AN
UNUSUAL COLLECTION OF
MEDICAL PERIODICAL SETS
MANY OF WHICH OF HISTORICAL
IMPORTANCE

FOLLOWED BY

A COLLECTION OF ABOUT 300
INTERNATIONAL CONGRESSES
ON MEDICAL SUBJECTS

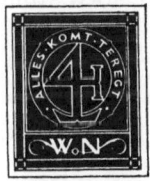

SPRINGER-SCIENCE+BUSINESS MEDIA, B.V.

Cable address: Books. - Adams Cable Cod. 10th ed. - Teleph. 110117

Prices are in Dutch guilders

1 guilder is about $ 0.55

My American customers may send their orders through Messrs TICE & LYNCH, forwarding agents, 21 Pearl Street, New York City.

ISBN 978-94-015-2159-8   ISBN 978-94-015-3371-3 (eBook)
DOI 10.1007/978-94-015-3371-3

Softcover reprint of the hardcover 1st edition 1939

MEDICAL PERIODICAL SETS

1. **Académie royale de médecine de Belgique.** Brux. 1841-1927. 115 vol. Av. pl. 4to et 8vo. br. et en livr.   800.—
La collection se compose comme suit:
   A. **Bulletin.** 1841-1927. Série 1-4, 5, t. 1-7. Av. tables génér. des séries 1-3. 78 vol.
   B. **Mémoires.** 1848-96. (Collection in-4to). 5 vol.
   Tout ce qui a paru.
   C. **Mémoires** des concours et des savants étrangers. (Collection in-4to). 1848-88. 8 vol.
   Tout ce qui a paru.
   D. **Mémoires** couronnés et autres mémoires. (Collection in-8vo). 1870-1926. T. 1-23. 23 vol.
   Ajouté: Cinquantième anniversaire de la fondation.
   C o l l e c t i o n   c o m p l è t e   d è s   l e   c o m m e n c e m e n t.   E x c e s s i v e m e n t   r a r e.

2. **Acta physico-medica Academica Caesareae-Leop.-Carolinae.** Norimb. 1737-54. T. 1-9. 9 vol. — **Nova Acta.** Norimb. 1757-83. T. 1-7. 7 vol. — Ens. 16 vol. Av. front. et pl. 4to. dont 9 vol. br., 7 cart.   100.—
3 vol. des ,,Acta" en 2e édition. Le titre du t. 6 des ,,Nova Acta" manque.
   Ajouté: **Miscellanea curiosa medico-physica** Acad. naturae curiosorum. Lps. 1670. Av. front. 4to. veau.

3. **Acta psychologica.** Ed. a G. Révész. H. C. 1936-39. T. 1-4. 4 vol. toile.   54.—
Revue internationale de psychologie. Parmi les collaborateurs nous citons: Fr. Ch. Bartlett, H. J. F. W. Brugmans, E. Claparède, A. Gemelli, P. Janet, K. S. Lashley, K. Marbe, M. Matsumoto, J. P. Pavlov, J. Piagèt, F. Roels, H. K. Schjelderup, W. Stern, R. M. Yerkes, e.a.
Chaque an un vol. de 400 pp. paraîtra. La première partie du t. I contient les ,,Papers read to the X. Internat. Congress of psychology, Copenhagen 1932" et comprend 232 pp. d'articles en français, en anglais et en allemand.

4.   — Idem. T. 1-4. 4 vol. En livr.   48.—

5. **Aesculaap.** Vaderlandsch tijdschrift voor theoretische en practische bijdragen in het gebied der genees-, heel- en verloskundige wetenschappen. Amst. 1835, 36. 2 vols.   15.—
All published.

6. **Annalen, Allgemeine medizinische.** Altenburg, Lpz. 1802, 1806-20, 1824-28. 25 vol. 4to. bound.   20.—
4 parts and 5 indexes missing.

7. **Annalen, Hannoversche,** für die gesammte Heilkunde. Hannover, 1838-46. Vol. 3-5; New series, vol. 1-6. 9 vols. In parts.   7.50
6 Indexes missing.

8. **Annalen, Heidelberger klinische.** Heidelberg, 1825–34. 10 vols. in 11. boards.   20.—
   All published.

9. **Annalen, Literarische,** der gesammten Heilkunde. Berlin u. Landsberg, 1825–35. Vol. 1–25, 29, 31. 27 vols. in 29. boards.   36.—
   Vol. 25 and ff. entitled: Wissenschaftl. u. neue wissenschaftl. Annalen. Titlepage, 5 indexes and 3 parts are missing.

10. **Annales des falsifications.** Bulletin internat. de la répression des fraudes alimentaires et pharmaceutiques. Réd. p. Ch. Franche et F. Touplain. Paris, 1908–29. Année 1–22. 22 tom. 21 vol. Av. pl. d. rel.   300.—
    Très rare et fort important.

11. **Annales de la médecine physiologique.** Paris, 1822–30. Vol. 1–17, 18, pp. 1–126. 17 vols. bound.   45.—

12. **Annales de la Société de médecine physique d'Anvers** (*plus tard*: **Annales de médecine physique et de physio–biologie**). Réd. Klynens; Gunzburg, e.a. Anvers, 1903–36. Année 1–29. Ens. 26 tom. 23 vol. Av. pl. dont 8 vol. d. rel., le reste en livr. *Très rare*.   225.—

13. **Annales de la Société de médecine de Gand.** Gand, 1835–1908. T. 1–88. — **Bulletin.** Gand, 1835–1908. T. 1–75. — Ens. 111 vol., dont 92 d. veau, le reste en livr.   300.—
    Annales, t. 63, 84 et 87 et Bulletin, t. 74 manquent.

14. **Annales de la Société de médecine de Lyon.** Lyon, 1896–1914. 2e Série, t. 44–55, 57–60. 16 vol. Av. pl.   60.—
    Ajouté: **Annales.** 2e Série, t 2, 2e sem., t. 13, 15, 22, 41. Lyon, 1854, 1867, 1874, 1893. — **Compte-rendu.** 1838.

15. **Annales pédologiques, Les.** Publ. par l'Institut national belge de pédologie. Brux. 1909–14. T. 1–4, 5, livr. 1–3. En livr.   20.—
    Tout ce qui a paru.

16. **Annual, The medical,** and practioner's index. Ed. by P. Wilde, A. G. Bateman, a.o. Bristol, 1887–1919. Année 5–37. 33 vol. Av. pl. et ill. toile (1 vol. cart.).   60.—

17. **Archief, Chemisch en pharmaceutisch.** Schoonhoven, 1840–42. 2 vols. bound.   10.—
    All published.

18. **Archief, Nederlandsch,** voor genees- en natuurkunde. Onder medewerk. van P. Q. Brondgeest, M. Imans, e.a. Uitgeg. d. F. C. Donders. Utrecht, 1865–70. 5 vol. Av. pl. cart.   35.—
    Collection complète.

19. **Archief, Nederlandsch militair-geneeskundig,** van de landmacht, zeemacht, het Oost en West Indische leger. Onder red. van J. H. Gentis en A. E. Post. Utrecht, 1877–97. T. 1–20. Av. pl. br. et en livr.   145.—
    Revue néerland. de médecine de l'armée et de la marine des Pays-Bas et des Indes Néerlandaises. Très rare.
    Les titres et les tables des tom. 17 et 20 manquent.

20. **Archief, Nieuw,** voor binnen- en buitenlandsche geneeskunde in haren geheelen omvang d. I. van Deen. Zwolle, 1845–51. Année 1–3, 4, livr. 1–3. 4 vol. Av. pl. d. rel.   12.50
    Collection complète.

21. **Archiv für Anatomie und Physiologie.** Lpz. 1826–28, 1832. Vol. 1–3, 6 (last vol. publ.). 4 vols. boards   24.—
    Year 1831 was never published.

Prices are in Dutch guilders

22. **Archiv für die Geburtshülfe, Frauenzimmer- und neugeborener Kinderkrankheiten** von J. C. Starke. Jena, 1787–1802. Vol. 1–6; New series, vol. 1, 2. 8 vols. W. pl. boards. 35.—
The last part (vol. 3, no. 1), publ. in 1804, is lacking.

23. **Archiv für Geschichte der Medizin.** Hrsg. v. d. Puschmann-Stiftung an der Universität Leipzig. Red. K. Sudhoff. Lpz. 1908–12. T. 1–6. 6 vol. Av. pl. et figg. En livr. 24.—
T. 6, livr. 6 manque.

24. **Archiv für Gynäkologie.** Hrsg. von F. Birnbaum, C. Braun u. A. Berlin, 1870–1932. T. 1–148. 148 vol. Av. tables des tom. 1–100. Ens. 149 vol. rel. 585.—

25. **Archiv der Heilkunde.** Lpz. 1860–78. 19 vols. boards. 35.—
All published.

26. **Archiv für die homoopatische Heilkunst.** Lpz. 1822–28. Vol. 1–6, 7, part 1, 2. 6 vols. 20.—

27. **Archiv für klinische Chirurgie.** Hrsg. von B. von Langenbeck, Th. Billroth, u. A. Berlin, 1861–1937. Vol. 1–188. W. indexes to vols. 1–100, 121–150. Tog. 190 vols. of which 162 hfcloth, 15 boards and 13 in parts. 800.—
2 pl. (in vol. 7 and 64) missing. Librarystamp on titlepages.

28. **Archiv für Laryngologie und Rhinologie.** Hrsg. von B. Fränkel. Berlin, 1902–14. T. 12–28, 29, livr. 1, 2. 18 tom. 15 vol. Av. pl. en couleurs et en noir. d. rel. unif. 90.—
En partie épuisé. Nom sur 3 titres, du reste en parfait état.

29. **— Idem.** Berlin, 1906–11, 19–25. 7 vol. Av. pl. En livr. 20.—

30. **Archiv für Ophthalmologie** von Graefe. Berlin u. Lpz. 1854–1908. Année 1–67. Av. table des années 1–50. 68 vol. Av. pl. d. veau unif. *Bel ex.* 450.—

31. **Archiv für pathologische Anatomie und Physiologie** und für klinische Medizin. Hrsg. von R. Virchow. Berlin, 1847–1919. T. 1–226. 226 vol. Av. tous les suppl. et tables des tom. 1–200. 237 vol. Av. pl. d. rel. unif. 1600.—
Plusieurs volumes sont de la réimpression.

32. **Archiv für physiologische Heilkunde.** Stuttgart, 1842–50. 15 vols.; New series, vol. 1–3. 18 vols. W. pl. boards. 40.—
All published. 2 titlepages and indexes missing.

33. **Archiv für Psychiatrie und Nervenkrankheiten.** Hrsg. von W. Griesinger, O. Bumke u.A. Berlin, 1868–1928, 1933–34. T. 1–83, 98–102. Av. suppl. du t. 22 et index des tom. 1–45. 90 vol. Av. pl. et ill. dont 53 vol. d. rel., le reste cart. 525.—

34. **— Idem.** Berlin, 1868–70. Vol. 1, 2. 2 vols. W. pl. boards. 7.50

35. **Archiv für Rassen- und Gesellschafts-Biologie** einschliessl. Rassen- und Gesellschafts-Hygiene. Hrsg. von A. Ploetz u. A. Berlin, 1904–29. Année 1–21. 21 tom. 20 vol. Av. pl. d. rel. 360.—
Tous les volumes en édition originale.

36. **Archiv für den thierischen Magnetismus.** Hrsg. von C. A. von Eschenmayer, D. G. Kieser und F. Nasse. Altenburg, 1817–24. 12 tom. 6 vol. d. rel. 120.—
Tout ce qui a paru de cet important périodique. Extrêmement rare en état complet.

37. **Archiv für Verdauungs-Krankheiten** mit Einschluss der Stoffwechselpathologie und der Diätetik. Red. von J. Boas. Mit Beiheften. Berlin, 1895–1932. T. 1–52. 52 vol. Av. tables des tom. 1–50. 2 vol. Ens. 54 vol., dont 17 d. veau, le reste en livr.   325.—

38. **Archiv des Vereins für wissenschaftl. Arbeiten zur Förderung der wissenschaftl. Heilkunde.** Göttingen, 1854–67. Vol. 1–6; New series, vol. 1–3. 9 vols. W. pl.   25.—
   All published.

39. **Archives du magnétisme animal**, publ. par d'Hénin de Cuvillers. Paris, 1820–23. 8 vol.   50.—
   Tout ce qui a paru. Très rare.

40. **Archives néerlandaises de phonétique expérimentale.** Réd. par F. J. J. Buytendijk, W. Einthoven, H. Zwaardemaker, e.a. La Haye, 1927–39. T. 1–15. 15 vol. Av. figg.   75.—

41. **Archives néerlandaises de physiologie de l'homme et des animaux.** Réd. par W. Einthoven, H. J. Hamburger, C. A. Pekelharing e.a. La Haye, 1916–38. T. 1–23. 23 vol. Av. pl. et figg. En livr. (345.—)
                                                                        245.—
   En partie épuisé.

42. **Archives provinciales de chirurgie.** Réd. M. Baudouin. Paris, 1892–95, 1901. T. 1–4, 10. 5 vol. Av. ill. d. rel.   20.—
   Dans les tom. 2 et 3 7 portraits de chirurgiens manquent; en outre les pp. 197 à 200 du t. 2 manquent.

43. **Archivo de pharmacia e sciencias accessorias da India Portugueza.** Red. pelo A. Gomes Roberto. Nova Goa, 1865–71. Year 2–8. 7 vols.
                                                                        50.—
   Extremely scarce. After vol. 8 this publication was discontinued.

44. **Argos, Medizinischer.** Lpz. 1839–45. Vol. 1–5. 5 vols. partly bound.
                                                                        10.—
   1 Part missing.

45. **Artz, De,** of geneesheer in aangename spectatoriale vertoogen. Amst. (1765–71), 1784. 6 vols. in 12. — Idem. Nalezing. Amst. 1773–84. 4 vols in 3. — Tog. 10 vols in 15. boards.   75.—
   All published. The edition of 1765–71 with new titlepage.

46. **Arzt, Der.** Eine medicin. Wochenschrift. Hamburg, 1759–64. 12 vol. Av. portrait. d. veau.   50.—
   Tout ce qui a paru. Les tom. 1–7 avec quelques piqûres.

47. **Beiträge zur chemischen Physiologie und Pathologie.** Hrsg. von Fr. Hofmeister. Brschw. 1902–04. T. 1–5. 5 vol. toile.   20.—

48. **Berichte und Arbeiten a. d. geburtshülflichgynaekolog. Klinik zu Giessen,** 1881–1886, von F. Ahlfeld. Lpz. 1883–87. 3 vol. Av. pl. d. rel.   10.—
   Collection complète.

49. **Bibliotheek, Natuur- en geneeskundige.** Uitgeg. d. E. Sandifort. 's-Grav. 1765–75. 11 vols. bound.   50.—
   All published.

50. **Bibliotheek, Nieuwe natuur- en geneeskundige.** Amst. 1774. Vol. 1. calf.   10.—
   All published.

51. **Bibliothek der praktischen Heilkunde.** Berlin, 1799–1824. Vol. 1–24, 35–52. 42 vols. in 21. boards.   40.—

52. **Bibliothek, Chirurgische.** Hrsg. von A. G. Richter. Göttingen, 1771–97. 15 vol. Av. 2 vol. de tables. Ens. 17 vol. Av. pl. pet. in-8vo. d. veau. (Rel. légèr. endomm.). 40.—
    Tout ce qui a paru. Les pp. 81 et ss. du t. 2, livr. 3 manquent.

53. **Bibliothek, Medizinische,** von J. T. Blumenbach. Göttingen, 1783–88. 3 vols. Hfcalf. 12.—
    All published.

54. **Bibliothek, Medizinische practische,** worin Nachrichten zur Ausübung der Heilkunde. Göttingen, 1775–80. 3 vols. sm. 8vo. Hfcalf. 12.—
    All published.

55. **Bladen, Geneeskundige,** uit kliniek en laboratorium. Uitgeg. d. M. Straub, H. Treub en W. Nolen. Haarlem, 1894–1921. T. 1–22. 22 vol., dont 1–18 d. rel. unif. (± 200.— br.) 90.—

56. **Bladen, Psychiatrische.** Red. Tellegen, Cowan en van Deventer. Dordrecht, 1883–96. 14 vol. cart. – **Psychiatrische en neurologische bladen.** Uitgeg. d. de Nederl. Vereeniging voor psychiatrie en neurologie. Red. Jelgersma e.a. Amst. 1897–1933. Année 1–37. 37 vol. toile orig. 250.—
    Série complète dès le commencement de l'organe de la Société néerland. de psychiatrie et de neurologie.

57. **Bladen, Psychiatrische en neurologische.** Uitgeg. d. de Nederl. Vereen. voor psychiatrie en neurologie. Red. G. Jelgersma, C. Bijl e.a. Amst. 1897–1928. Année 1–32. 32 vol. Av. pl. et figg. dont 10 vol. toile, 14 cart., 8 en livr. 165.—
    Les nos. 3 à 6 du ,,Bijblad" du t. 32 n'existent pas.

58. **Boerhave.** Tijdschrift voor genees-, heel-, verlos- en artsenymengkunde. Amst., 's-Grav. 1838–48. 10 vols. W. pl. bound. 45.—
    All published.

59. **Bulletin de l'Académie de médecine.** Paris, 1872–85. 2e Série, t. 1–14. Av. figg. cart. 20.—
    2 titres manquent.

60. **Bulletin des sciences physiques et naturelles en Néerlande.** Réd. par F. A. W. Miquel, G. J. Mulder, e.a. Leiden, 1839, 40. 2 vols. W. pl. bound. 15.—
    All published.

61. **Bulletin de la Société médicale de l'Yonne,** 1860–1923/24. Auxerre, 1862–1925. T. 1–59. 59 vol. Av. ill. 290.—

62. **Bijdragen tot de theoretische en practische geneeskunde.** Amst. 1810–13. Vol. 1, 2, 3, part 1. 10.—
    All published. 1 Index and 2 parts missing.

63. **Bijdragen, Geneeskundige,** d. C. Pruys van der Hoeven. Delft, Rott. 1825–30. 3 vols. 15.—
    All published.

64. **Centralblatt für allgem. Gesundheitspflege.** Organ des Niederrhein. Vereins für öffentl. Gesundheitspflege. Bonn, 1882–99. Année 1–6, 12, 18. Ens. 10 vol. toile. 20.—

65. **Centralblatt für allgem. Pathologie und patholog. Anatomie.** Hrsg. von E. Ziegler. Jena, 1890–1914. T. 1–25. Av. table des tom. 1–20. 26 vol. Av. pl. en couleurs et en noir. toile. *Bel ex., bien relié.* 300.—

66. **Centralblatt für Gynäkologie.** Hrsg. von H. Fehling und H. Fritsch. Lpz. 1885–1909. T. 9–33. 25 vol. d. veau unif.   55.—

67. **Centralblatt, Internat.,** für Laryngologie, Rhinologie und verwandte Wissenschaften. Hrsg. von F. Semon. Berlin, 1899–1900, 1905–11. Année 15, 16, 21–27. 9 vol. d. rel.   28.—

68. **Centralblatt, Internat.,** für die Physiologie und Pathologie der Harn- und Sexual-Organe. Hrsg. von W. Zuelzer. Hamburg, Lpz. 1889–1906. Year 1–17. 17 vols. — (*Continued by:*) **Zeitschrift für Urologie.** Red. L. Casper, A. von Frisch, u. A. Lpz. 1907–21. Vol. 1–15. 15 vols. — Tog. 32 vols. of which 1–17 hfcalf, the remainder sewed.   225.—

69. **Centralblatt, Neurologisches.** Uebersicht der Leistungen a.d. Gebiete der Anatomie, Physiologie, Pathologie und Therapie des Nerven-systems einschliessl. der Geisteskrankheiten. Hrsg. von E. Mendel. Lpz. 1895–1919. Année 14–38. 25 vol. d. rel. unif. (1919 en livr.).   100.—

70. **Centralzeitung, Berliner medicin.** Berlin, 1832–91. Year 1–60. 53 vols. 4to and fol. boards.   85.—
Year 13–18 are missing.

71. **Cholera, De.** Bijblad tot de Geneeskundige courant voor het Kon. der Nederlanden. Tiel, 1 Julij–9 Dec. 1849. 23 nos. cart.   7.50
Tout ce qui a paru.

72. **Commentaries, Medical.** Edinburgh, 1787–92. 2d series, vol. 1–6. 6 vols.   10.—

73. **Conseil supérieur d'hygiène publique.** Rapports au Ministre de l'Intérieur, 1849–1915. Brux. 1856–1916. T. 1–20. 20 vol. d. veau.   82.50

74. **Correspondenz-Blatt für Schweizer Aerzte.** Hrsg. von E. Klebs, A. Burckhardt-Merian, A. Baader u. A. Bern, Basel, 1871–1927. Année 1–57. 57 vol. Av. pl. gr. in-8vo et gr. in-4to. dont 5 vol. d. veau, 28 d. rel., 9 cart., le reste en livr.   250.—
Année 50–57 sous le titre: Schweizerische medizinische Wochenschrift. Hrsg. von E. Hedinger u. P. Von der Mühll. 5 vol. gr. in-4to.

75. **Dentistry.** — **Ash's Wiener Vierteljahrs-Fachblatt.** Neues und Wissenswertes a. d. zahnärztl. und zahntechnischen Gebiete. Wien, 1905–13. Year 1–9. 9 vols. hfcloth.   45.—

76. — **Correspondenzblatt für Zahnärzte.** Berlin, 1872–1937. Year 1–60, 61, part 1–6. 61 vols in 60, of which 57 bound, the remainder in parts.   350.—
Vol. 7, no. 4 and several titles and indexes are missing.

77. — **Cosmos, The dental.** A monthly record of dental science. Philadelphia, 1860–1936. Vol. 1–78. bound in 114 vols. hfcloth.   350.—

78. — **Ergebnisse der gesamten Zahnheilkunde.** Hrsg. Von G. Fischer u. A. Wiesbaden, 1911–24. Vol. 1–7. 7 vols. W. pl. hfcloth.   32.—

79. — **Fortschritte, Die,** der Zahnheilkunde. Lpz. 1925–33. Vol. 1–9. 18 vols. bound.   120.—

80. — **Journal, The American,** of dental science. N.-York, 1839–55. 1st Series, 9 vols; New series, vol. 1–5. Tog. 14 vols. bound in 13. hfcalf.   150.—

Prices are in Dutch guilders

81. **Dentistry. — Lapja, Magyar Fogorvosik.** Ed. J. Antal. Budapest, 1906–07. 2 vols. — (*Continued by:*) **Fogorvosi Szemle.** Ed. Z. Körmöczi and G. Morelli. Budapest, 1908–march 1938. Vol. 1–30, 31, part 1–3. W. pl. and ill. 32 vols. in 22. 275.—
Journal of the Hungarian stomatological Association.
Missing: Vol. 12 (1919, if publ.); vol. 29, part 9; vol. 30, part 5; titles of several vols. (if ever publ.) and several pp., contain. advertisements only.

82. **— Odontoskop.** Magyar Fogaszati Folyoirat. Ed. J. Iszlai. Budapest, 1892–97. 5 years. bound in 2 vols. 50.—
All published. Title and index of year 5 are missing (if ever publ.).

83. **— Revue (mensuelle) de stomatologie.** Paris, 1900–14. Year 7–20, 21, nos. 1–7. 15 vols. bound. 100.—

84. **— Verhandlungen der deutschen odontolog. Gesellschaft.** Berlin, 1890–95. T. 1–6. 3 vol. Av. pl. cart. *Rare.* 30.—

85. **— Vierteljahrsschrift, Deutsche,** für Zahnheilkunde. Wien, 1861-82. 22 vols. — (*Continued by:*) **Deutsche Monatsschrift für Zahnheilkunde.** Berlin, 1883–1933. Year 1–51. — Tog. 73 vols. in 75 of which 10 hfcalf, the remainder hfcloth. 600.—
Missing: Vol. 6, part 3, pp. 161–244; vol. 8, pp. 213–220.

86. **— — Idem.** 1861–1913. Vol. 1–31. 51 vols., of which 48 bound. 450.—
Vol. 6 and 8 of Vierteljahrsschrift are missing.

87. **— Vierteljahrsschrift, Oesterreichisch-Ungarische,** für Zahnheilkunde. Wien, 1885–1918. Year 1–34. — (*Continued by:*) **Wiener Vierteljahrsschrift für Zahnheilkunde.** Wien, 1919–20. Year 35–36; — (*Continued by:*) **Vierteljahrsschrift für Zahnheilkunde.** Berlin, 1921–33. Year 37–49. — Tog. 49 vols. hfcloth. 600.—
6 pp. in vol. 16 and 18 damaged; some other pp. are missing, containing advertisements only.

88. **— Vierteljahrsschrift, Schweizerische,** für Zahnheilkunde. (Revue trimestrielle suisse d'odontologie). Zürich, 1895–1921. Vol. 5-31. 27 vols. — (*Continued by:*) **Schweizerische Monatsschrift für Zahnheilkunde.** Zürich, 1922–37. Vol. 32–47. 16 vols. Tog. 43 vols. hfcloth. 425.—
Some pp. in several vols., containing advertisements only, are missing.

89. **— Zahnarzt, Der.** Das Neueste und Wissenswürdigste des In- und Auslandes über Zahnheilkunde. Berlin, 1846–72. 27 vols. bound. (Some bindings broken). 125.—
All published.
Missing: Vol. 20, nos. 10–12; vol. 22, no. 4; vol. 27, pp. 115–126; 3 pl. and one index. Some „Beilagen" are also missing, but they contain advertisements only.

90. **— Zeitschrift, Österreichische,** für Stomatologie — (*later:* **Zeitschrift für Stomatologie**). Red. G. von Wunschheim u. A. Berlin, Wien, 1907–37. Year 5–35. 31 vols. W. pl. hfcloth. 400.—

91. **Ellenberger-Schütz' Jahresbericht über die Leistungen a. d. Gebiete der Veterinär-Medizin.** Hrsg. von W. Ellenberger, K. Neumann-Kleinpaul u. O. Zietzschmann. Berlin, 1921–26. Année 38–44. 5 vol. 125.—
En partie épuisé.

92. **Essays, Medical,** and observations publ. by a society in Edinburgh. Edinburgh, 1752. 6 vols. W. pl. sm. 8vo. calf. 15.—

93. **Excerpta medica.** Kurze monatliche Journalauszüge a.d. gesammten Fachlitteratur. Hrsg. von E. Graetzer. Lpz. 1891–1905. Année 1–14. 14 vol. En livr.   15.—

94. **Flandre médicale, La,** (*plus tard*: La Belgique médicale). Revue scientifique et pratique. Publ. par A. Claus, D. de Buck, e.a. Gand, 1894–98. Année 1–5. 9 vol. En livr.   20.—
   Le no. 38 de l'année 3 manque.

95. **Food journal, The.** Social and sanitary economy and monthly record of food and public. London, 1870–73. 4 vols. boards.   10.—
   All published. 1 titlepage and index missing.

96. **Gazette, The monthly,** of health. London, 1816–22. Vol. 1–7. 7 vols.
                                                                       7.50
   2 titlepages and 1 index missing.

97. **Geist und Kritik** der medicin. und chirurg. Zeitschriften Deutschlands. Lpz. 1798–1806. 9 vols. in 18.   45.—
   All published.

98. **Handelingen** van het geneeskundig genootschap Servandibus Civibus. Amst. 1776–92. 15 vols. in 18. boards.   70.—
   All published.

99. **l'Hermès.** Journal du magnétisme animal. Par une société de médecins. Paris, 1826–29. 4 tom. 2 vol. d. veau.   45.—
   Tout ce qui a paru. Très rare.

99a. **Hippocrate.** Revue d'humanisme médical. Dir.: Laignel-Lavastine. Paris, 1933–37. Année 1–5. 5 vol. Av. pl. et ill. dont 1 vol. toile, couv. cons., le reste en livr.   40.—

100. **Hippocrates.** Magazijn toegewijd aan de geneeskunde. Amst. 1813–37. Vol. 1–7, 8, part 1, 2. 8 vols. W. pl.   56.—
   All published.

101. **Hoefsmid, De.** Geïll. maandblad voor hoefsmeden e. a. die in het hoefbeslag belangstellen. Red. A. W. Heidema e.a. Groningen, 's-Grav. 1896–1926. Année 1–31. 31 vol. Av. pl. et ill. dont 19 vol. toile, le reste en livr.   40.—

102. **Hufschmied, Der.** Zeitschrift für das gesammte Hufbeschlagswesen. Red. von A. Lungwitz. Dresden, 1895–1916. Année 13–34. 22 vol. Av. ill. et figg. dont 20 vol. d. rel., le reste en livr.   18.—
   Le no. 5 de l'année 30 manque. Ajoutée l'année 4. Dresden, 1886.

103. **Hygiea.** Medicinsk och farmaceutisk Månadsskrift. Stockholm, 1839–1929. Year 1–91. W. index of the years 1839–1920 and 2 „Festalbum". Year 1839–1860 in 22 vols. boards, 1861–1911 in 80 vols. unif. hfbound, the remainder in parts.   290.—

104. **Jaarboek, Paedologisch.** Uitgeg. d. h. stedelijke gemeentebestuur (van Antwerpen) onder red. van M. C. Schuÿten. Antw. 1900–04. Année 1–5. En 4 vol. Av. pl.   20.—
   Tout ce qui a paru. Presque tous les articles sont accompagnées d'un résumé en langue française ou anglaise.

105. **Jaarboeken der genees-, heel- en natuurkunde.** Amst. 1812–18. 4 vols. W. pl. In parts.   20.—
   All published. 1 Part missing.

106. **Jaarboeken, Genees-, natuur- en huishoudkundige.** Dordrecht, Amst. 1778–82. 13 vols. — **Jaarboeken, Nieuwe.** Ib. 1782–84. 10 vols. — Tog. 23 vols. boards.   60.—
   All published.

Prices are in Dutch guilders

107. **Jahrbuch der Radioaktivität und Elektronik.** Unter Mitarbeit von S. A. Arthenius, P. und S. Curie, H. A. Lorentz u. A. hrsg. von J. Stark und R. Seeliger. Lpz. 1904–23. T. 1–20. 20 vol. Av. pl. et ill. dont 17 vol. cart., le reste en livr. 225.—
Tout ce qui a paru. Uni avec le Physikalische Zeitschrift.

108. **Jahrbuch der Staatsarzneikunde** von Kopp. Frankfurt, 1808–19. Vol. 1–10, 11, part 1, 2. 11 vols. W. pl. boards. 20.—
All published.

109. **Jahrbücher der Medicin als Wissenschaft.** Tübingen, 1806–07. Vol. 1, 2. 2 vols. bound. 7.50

110. **Jahrbücher der Teutschen Medicin und Chirurgie.** Nürnberg, 1813. 3 vols. — *(Continued by:)* **Rheinische Jahrbücher der Medicin und Chirurgie.** Bonn, 1819–26. 12 vols. — Tog. 15 vols. W. pl. bound. 70.—
All published. 2 Indexes missing.

111. **Jahrbücher, Medicinische,** des K. K. Oesterreich. Staates. Wien, 1822–44. T. 7–50. Av. ,,Ergänzungsblatt: **Oesterreich. medicin. Wochenschrift"**, 1841–1844. Ens. 43 vol. Av. pl. cart. 65.—
Manquent du t. 16, 1 pl., du t. 30, les pp. 337—352 et 1 pl. et du ,,Wochenschrift", la table de 1842 et les pp. 641–644 de 1844, I. Marque de bibliothèque sur les titres.

112. **Jahrbücher, Medizinische,** der K. K. Geselschaft der Aerzte in Wien, 1861–1883. Wien, 1861–83. 25 vols. 4to. boards. 48.—
Set from the beginning. This periodical was discontinued in 1888.

113. **Jahresbericht über die Fortschritte in der Lehre von den pathogenen Mikroorganismen,** umfassend Bacterien, Pilze und Protozoën. Hrsg. von P. Baumgarten u. W. Dibbelt. Brschw. u. Lpz. 1886–1917. 27 tom. 40 vol. Av. tables des tom. 1–10. 110.—
Collection complète.

114. **Janus.** Archives pour l'histoire de la médecine et la géographie médicale. Réd. en chef H. F. A. Peypers, e.a. Harlem, etc. 1896–1931. Année 1–35. Av. table des années 1895–1905. 35 vol. Av. pl. dont 28 vol. cart., 7 en livr. 600.—
Très recherché.

115. **Journal de l'anatomie et de la physiologie normales** et pathologiques de l'homme et des animaux. Paris, 1864–75. Vol. 1–11. 11 vols. W. pl. boards. 40.—
1 Titlepage missing.

116. **Journal de chimie médicale, de pharmacie et de toxicologie.** Paris, 1825–26, 32–36. T. 1, 2, 8–10; 2e Série, t. 1, 2. 7 vol. Av. pl. d. veau. 5.— per vol.
Ajouté: Le même. Paris, 1843, 44. 2e série, t. 9, nos 2—3, 5, 7—8, 11; t. 10, nos 3—4, 6—7, 9—12. En livr. 1.— per livr.

117. **Journal für die Chirurgie, Geburtshülfe und gerichtliche Arzneikunde.** Jena, 1797–1806. 4 vols. W. pl. bound. 12.50
All published.

118. **Journal of comparitive pathology and therapeutics.** Edinburgh, 1891. T. 4. En livr. *Rare.* 18.—

119. **Journal des connaissances médico-chirurgicales** — *(later:* **Revue de thérapeutique médico-chirurgicale**). Paris, 1837, 1850–62. Year 5, 17–20. 14 vols. W. ill. boards. 10.—

10 MEDICAL PERIODICAL SETS

120. **Journal für Kinderkrankheiten.** Berlin und Erlangen, 1843–72.
59 vols. W. index to vol. 1–31. In 61 vols.   120.—
All published.
Slightly stained by water without damaging the text.

121. **Journal du magnétisme.** Par une Société de magnétiseurs et
de médecins sous la dir. de du Potet. Paris, 1845–61. 20 tom. 17
vol. d. veau.   100.—
Tout ce qui a paru. Très rare.

122. **Journal de médecine,** ou observat. des plus fameux médecins,
chirurgiens et anatomistes de l'Europe, tirées des journaux des
pais étrangers, et des mémoires particuliers envoyéz à l'abbé de
La Roque. Paris, 1683. W. 2 pl. sm. 8vo. calf.   40.—
One of the oldest medical periodicals. It contains i.a. letters from
Leeuwenhoek on his microscopical discoveries (pp. 112–128 and 203–222,
w. 2 engrav.).
Exceedingly scarce. This is the first volume, only 3 more are known.
Bound up with: **Dionis,** Histoire anatomique d'une matrice extraordi-
naire. Paris, 1683. W. 1 (instead of 2) pl.

123. **Journal de pharmacie.** Publ. par la Société de pharmacie d'Anvers.
Dir. Acar, Molyn, e.a. Anvers, 1845–1914. 70 années. — **Annales
de pharmacie.** Publ. p. F. Ranwez. Louvain, 1895–1914. 20 années.
— *(Réunis et continués comme:)* **Journal de pharmacie de Belgique.**
Brux. 1919–30. Année 1–12. — Ens. 102 tom. 101 vol. Av. pl.
d. rel.   800.—
Collection complète (de 1915–1918 rien n'a paru), excessivement rare.

124. **Journal für Pharmakodynamik, Toxicologie und Therapie.** Berlin,
1856, 60. 2 vols. boards.   10.—
All published.

125. **Journal de la physiologie de l'homme et des animaux.** Paris, 1858–
63. 6 vols. W. pl. boards.   50.—
All published.

126. **Journal des sciences médicales de Louvain.** Louvain, 1876–81.
6 vol. — *(Continué par:)* **Revue médicale.** Louvain, 1882–1903.
19 vol. — *(Continué par:)* **Revue médicale de Louvain.** Année
1904–1930. Louvain, 1904–30. 24 tom. 23 vol. — Ens. 49 tom.
48 vol., dont 27 vol. d. veau, 19 d. rel., 2 en livr.   335.—

127. **Journal médical de la Néerlande.** La Haye, 1844. Vol. 1, nr. 1–11.
                                                           10.—
All published.

128. **Journal universel et hebdomadaire de médecine et de chirurgie
pratique.** Paris, 1830–33. Vol. 1–12. 12 vols. W. pl. boards. 20.—
9 Indexes are missing (if published). The last volume published (vol. 13)
is lacking.

129. **Journal, The American,** of the medical sciences. N. York, Philadelphia, 1828–35, 1857–69. Nos. 2–32; New Series, vols. 33–51,
53–58. 39 vols. boards.   120.—
Titlepages to the first series are missing (published?).

130. **Kabinet, Genees-, natuur- en huishoudkundig.** Leiden, 1781, 82.
Vol. 2, 3. 4 vols. W. pl. boards.   7.50

131. **Kliniek.** Tijdschrift voor wetenschappelijke geneeskunde. Utrecht,
1844–49. 4 vols.   15.—
All published. 6 pp. and 1 index missing.

Prices are in Dutch guilders

132. **Klinik, Wiener.** Vorträge aus der gesammten pract. Heilkunde. Red. von J. Schnitzler u. A. Bum. Wien, 1875–91. Année 1–17. 17 vol. Av. ill., dont 12 vol. toile et d. rel., le reste en livr. 12.—

133. **Lancet, Het.** Maandschrift voor practische genees-, heel- en verloskunde. Tiel, 1860–78. 1re Série, 8 vol.; N. S., année 1–11. Ens. 19 vol., dont 3 vol. d. veau, 10 d. rel., le reste en feuilles. 40.—
   N. S., année 6, livr. 9 manque.

134. **Leistungen und Fortschritte, Die,** der Medicin in Deutschland. Berlin, 1833–36. 5 vols. — **Jahrbuch für die Leistungen der gesammten Heilkunde.** Lpz. 1837–42. 10 vols. — Tog. 15 vols. boards. 50.—
   All published. The index of year 10, part 1, 2 missing (not published?).

135. **Leven, Het toekomstig.** Halfmaandelijksch tijdschrift gewijd aan de studie der proefondervindelijke zielkunde (spiritisme) en bovenaardsche verschijnselen. Utrecht, etc. 1897–1927. Année 1–31. 31 vol. 4to. dont 1–21 toile orig., le reste en livr. 60.—
   Le „Future Life" hollandais.

136. **Light.** Journal of psycholog. occult and mystical research. London, 1900–19. T. 20–39. 20 vol. fol. dont 1900–1912 en 13 vol. d. rel., le reste en livr. 25.—
   Les nos. 1739 et 1802 et les titres et tables des années 1909, 1916 et 1919 manquent.

137. **Literatur, Medicinische,** für practische Aerzte. Lpz. 1781–87. 12 vols. — **Neue medicinische Literatur** für practische Aerzte. Lpz. 1787–92. Vol. 1–4. 4 vols. — Tog. 16 vols. in 10. Hfcalf and boards. 45.—
   All published.

138. **Loire médicale, La.** St. Etienne, 1891–1902. Année 10–21. 12 tom. Av. pl. En 8 vol. d. rel. 15.—
   Très rare. 10 numéros et une partie des titres manquent.

139. **Lucina.** Zeitschrift zur Vervollkommnung der Entbindungskunst. Lpz. 1802–09. 6 vols. in 3. boards. 15.—
   All published.

140. **Maandblad voor apothekers** gewijd aan de wetenschappelijke belangen der pharmacie. Red. H. van Geldcr, e.a. Gorinchem, 1887–88. d. rel. 5.—
   Revue mensuelle néerland. des apothécaires. Collection complète.

141. **Maandschrift, Nederlandsch,** voor verloskunde en vrouwenziekten en voor kindergeneeskunde. Red. P. C. T. van der Hoeven en G. Scheltema (*depuis l'année IX*: Nederl. maandschrift voor geneeskunde). Leiden, 1912–24. Année 1–12. 12 vol. Av. pl. et figg. toile. 65.—

142. **Magazin für die gesammte Heilkunde.** Berlin, 1816–47. Vol. 1–52, 57–60, 64–66, nrs. 1–2 (last published). 44 vols. 35.—
   Missing 2 parts and 3 titlepages and indexes.

143. **Magazin der ausländischen Literatur der gesammten Heilkunde.** Hamburg, 1821–35. 20 vols; New series, 10 vols. — (*Continued by:*) **Zeitschrift für die gesammte Medicin** mit besond. Rücksicht auf Hospitalpraxis. Hamburg, 1836–51. 45 vols. — Tog. 76 vols. boards. 100.—
   All published. 2 parts missing.

144. **Magazin zur Vervollkommnung der theoretischen und practischen Heilkunde.** Frankfurt, 1799–1807. 10 vols. sm. 8vo. boards. 60.—
All published.

145. **Magazijn, Geneeskundig.** Delft en Leiden, 1801–15. 5 vols. in 7. bound. Hfcalf. 35.—
All published. 2 indexes missing.

146. **Meddelanden, Oto-laryngologiska.** Utg. af G. Holmgren. Stockholm, 1912–16. T. 1, 2. 2 vol. Av. pl. et figg. En livr. 6.— per vol.

147. **Mededeelingen van den Burgerlijken Geneeskundigen Dienst** (*plus tard*: Dienst der volksgezondheid) **in Nederl.-Indië.** Onder red. van P. H. Olivier, E. R. K. Rodenwaldt e.a. Batavia, 1912–39. Année 1–27, 28, no. 1. ± 100 vol. et fasc. Av. cartes et pl. en couleurs et en noir et figg. cart. et br. 290.—
Publications du service médical des Indes Néerlandaises, conten. des contributions intéressantes de N. H. Swellengrebel, P. C. Flu, W. A. Borger, C. D. de Langen, L. Otten, P. H. M. Travaglino, S. L. Brug, B. C. P. Jansen, e.a. en langues néerland., anglaise ou allemande.
Année 1924, t. 2 contient: **L. Otten,** De pest op Java, 1911–1923. 144 pp. Av. cartes, ill. et tabl.

148. **Mededeelingen uit het geneeskundig laboratorium te Weltevreden.** Batavia, 1901–20. 2e Série A, nos. 2–17; 2e Série B, nos. 2–10; 3e Série A, t. 1–4. Av. pl. 8vo et 4to. En livr. 75.—
Série complète très rare des communications du Laboratoire médical à Weltevreden (Java) (en partie en deux langues: néerland. et anglais ou allemand). Les volumes précédents ont paru dans le ,,Indisch tijdschrift voor geneeskunde''.

149. **Mémoires de l'Académie Royale de chirurgie.** Paris, 1743–74. 5 vol. Av. pl. 4to. veau. 45.—
Collection complète.

150. **Mémoires de la Société médicale d'émulation de Lyon.** Lyon, 1842. T. 1. *Rare.* 7.50

151. **Mémoires de la Société médicale d'émulation de Paris.** Paris, 1798–1826. 9 vol. Av. pl. d. veau. 65.—
Tout ce qui a paru.

152. **Mémoires et comptes-rendus de la Société des sciences médicales de Lyon.** Lyon, 1880–96. T. 19–35. 17 vol. 30.—

153. **Mengelingen, Geneeskundige.** Amst. 1820, 24. 2 vols. W. pl. 18.—
All published.

154. **Mitteilungen über allgem. Pathologie und patholog. Anatomie der Kaiserl. Universität zu Sendai, Japan.** Sendai, 1921–28. T. 1–4, 5, livr. 1. 5 vol. Av. pl. En livr. 40.—
T. 1, livr. 1 manque.

155. **Mittheilungen a.d. gynaekolog. Klinik des Prof. Dr. Otto Engström in Helsingfors.** Berlin, 1897–1911. T. 1–9. Av. ,,Festschrift Engström''. Ens. 10 vol. Av. pl. en couleurs. d. rel. unif. 24.—

156. **Monatshefte, Therapeutische.** Hrsg. von O. Liebreich. Berlin, 1887–1921. 35 vol. dont 11 vol. d. rel., le reste en livr. 90.—
Collection complète. Continué par Klinische Wochenschrift.

157. **Monatsschrift für Geburtshilfe und Gynaekologie.** Red. von A. Martin und M. Sänger. Berlin, 1895–1907. T. 1–26. Av. ,,Ergänzungsheft zu Bd V'' et tables des tom. 1–35. Ens. 29 vol. Av. pl. en couleurs et en noir. d. veau unif. 65.—

158. **Monatsschrift für Ohrenheilkunde** sowie für Kehlkopf, Nasen-, Rachen-Krankheiten. Hrsg. von J. Gruber, J. M. Rossbach, u. A. Berlin, 1893–1917. Année 27–51. 25 vol. Av. pl. En livr. 70.—

159. **Monatschrift, Schweizerische,** für praktische Medizin. Hrsg. von Bellmont und A. Vogt. Bern, 1856–60. 5 vol. Av. pl. cart. 24.—
Tout ce qui a paru.

160. **Moniteur d'hygiène** et de salubrité publique, domestique, agricole, industrielle. Publ. par A. Chevallier. Paris, 1866–69. 4 vols. boards. 15.—
All published. Merged into Journal de chimie médicale. Titlepages to vol. 3 and 4 are missing (if published).

161. **Montpellier médical.** Journal mensuel de médecine. Montpellier, 1859–67. T. 2–15, 17–19. 17 vol. Av. pl. d. veau (2 dos endomm.). 50.—
Le titre du t. III manque.

162. **Museum, The medical,** or a repository of cases, experiments, researches and discoveries. London, 1763–64. 3 vols. Hfcalf. 12.—
All published.

163. **Nachrichten, Medicinische und chirurgische Berlinische wöchentliche.** Berlin, 1742–52. 6 vols. 4to. 30.—
All published.

164. **Notizen a.d. Gebiete der Natur- und Heilkunde.** Weimar, 1834–36. Vol. 41–50. In 5 vols. 4to. — (*Continued by:*) **Neue Notizen,** u.s.w. Weimar, 1837–49. 40 vols.; 3d series 11 vols. Tog. in 28 vols. 4to. — **Froriep's Tagsberichte** über die Fortschritte der Natur- und Heilkunde. Weimar, 1850–53. 8 vols. — **Notizen, Neue Fortsetzung.** Weimar, 1856–62. Year 1–7 in 13 vols. 4to. — Tog. 54 vols. 4to and 8vo (13 vols bound). 50.—
Missing: Froriep's Tagsberichte 1853 and 15 titlepages and 14 indexes.

165. **Organ für die gesammte Heilkunde.** Bonn, 1840–42. Vol. 1, 2. 2 vols. W. pl. bound and sewed. 9.—
All published. 1 Titlepage and index missing.

166. **Practitioner, The independant.** Monthly journal devoted to medicine, surgery, obstetrics, dentistry, etc. N. York, 1884–88. T. 5–9. 5 vol. d. rel. 7.50

167. **Radium, Le.** La radioactivité et les radiations, les sciences qui s'y rattachent et leurs applications. Réd. J. Danne. Paris, 1904–19. 11 vol. Av. pl. et figg. En livr. 165.—
Tout ce qui a paru. Très rare.

168. **Recueil des sciences médicales.** Ypres, 1821–22. Vol. 1, 2, part. 1–8; 3, part 1–6. 3 vols. 4.—
2 Indexes missing.

169. **Recueil des travaux du Comité** consultatif d'hygiène publique de France. Paris, 1872–1905. Vol. 1–35. W. index to vols. 1–30. Tog. 32 vols. W. pl. 45.—

170. **Recueil périodique d'observations de médecine,** de chirurgie et de pharmacie. Paris, 1754–57. 7 vols. W. pl. calf. 30.—

171. **Répertoire annuel de clinique médico-chirurgicale.** Paris, 1833–40. 6 vols. cloth. 15.—
All published.

172. **Répertoire médico-chirurgical et obstétrical.** Brux. 1836–37. T.
1–4. 4 vols. Hfcalf. (Bindings damaged).   10.—
All published?

173. **Repertorium, Allgemeines,** der gesammten deutschen medicin.,
chirurg. Journalistik. Lpz. 1839–47. Year 13–21 (last publ.).
9 vols. 4to.   10.—
Missing: 1841, part 3; 1842, part 2, 3.

174. **Repertorium, Het.** Tijdschrift voor de geneeskunde in al haren
omvang. Amersfoort, Leiden, 1847–56. 7 vols. 4to; N. Series, vol.
1, 2. 8vo. Tog. 9 vols. bound.   35.—
All published.

175. **Repertorium, Kritisches,** für die gesammte Heilkunde. Berlin,
1823–33. 32 vols. W. index to vol. 1–30. 3 vols. Tog. 35 vols.
boards.   65.—
All published.

176. **Report of the medical officer of health** (Ch. Porter) on the public
health and sanitary circumstances of Johannesburg during 1st July,
1904–30 June, 1906. W. append. report by the medical attendant
(P. G. Stock) on the health of the natives and Indians employed
by the Council. Johannesburg, 1906. Av. pl. et tabl. fol.   7.50

177. **Reports of the sleeping sickness commissions.** London, 1903–12.
Nos. 1–12. 12 fasc. Av. pl. en couleurs et en noir.   25.—

178. **Review, The British and foreign medico-chirurgical,** or quarterly
journal of practical medicine and surgery. London, 1848–52.
Nos. 1–20. 20 vol.   20.—
Marque de bibliothèque sur les titres.

179. **Revue de chirurgie.** Dir. Ollier, Lejars, Quénu e. a. Paris, 1881–
1930. T. 1–68 vol. Av. pl. et figg. dont 46 vol. cart., le reste en
livr.   400.—

180. **Revue de gynécologie et de chirurgie abdominale.** Dir. S. Pozzi.
Paris, 1897–1913. T. 1–21. 21 vol. Av. pl. et figg. dont 18 vol. d.
veau, 3 en livr.   80.—

181. **Revue d'hygiène et de police sanitaire.** Réd. E. Vallin. Paris,
1879–1914. Année 1–35, 36, livr. 1–7. 35 vol. d. veau (et 7 livr.).
Bel ex.   170.—

182. **Revue spirite.** Journal d'études psychologiques et du spiritualisme
expérimental. Publ. p. A. Kardec. Paris, 1858–90. Année 1–33.
33 vol. d. chagr. vert, plats en toile. *Bel ex.*   60.—
La revue la plus documentée des revues sur le spiritisme.
Quelques titres et 3 tables manquent.

183. **Revue, Medische.** Maandelijksch overzicht der binnen- en buitenlandsche literatuur v. d. practiseerende geneesheer. Uitgeg. d. G.
C. Nijhoff, E. J. Buning, D. H. van der Goot e.a. Haarlem, 1901–
13. 13 vol. dont 11 vol. rel. et cart., le reste en livr.   40.—
Collection complète.

184. **Rivista sperimentale di freniatria e medicina legale delle aliènazioni
mentali.** Dir. A. Tamburini. Reggio-Emilia, 1909–13. T. 35–39.
5 vol. Av. pl. et figg. d. rel.   24.—

185. **Sammlung klinischer Vorträge.** Hrsg. von R. Volkmann. —
Gynaecologie. Nos. 1–104; N. F., nos. 1–174. — **Innere Medicin.** Nos. 1–118; N. F., nos. 1–143. — **Chirurgie.** Nos. 1–111;

Prices are in Dutch guilders

N. F., nos. 1–140. — Lpz. 1870–1908. 24 vol. toile, le reste en livr.
45.—

186. **Sammlung, Neue,** auserlesener Abhandlungen zum Gebrauche practischer Aerzte. Lpz. 1826–29. New Series, Vol. 2–12. 11 vols., 9 of which bound. 15.—

187. **Semaine médicale, La.** Réd. De Maurans. Paris, 1891–1914. Année 11–34 (dernier vol. publié). 24 vol. gr. in-4to. d. rel. 50.—

188. **Syphilidologie** oder die neuesten Erfahrungen, Beobachtungen und Fortschritte des Inlandes und Auslandes über die Erkenntniss und Behandlung der venerischen Krankheiten. Hrsg. von F.J.Behrend. Lpz., Erlangen, 1839–62. 7 vols.; New series, vol. 1–3. Tog. 10 vols. of which 4 bound. 60.—
Complete collection. In the years 1846–1857 nothing was published.

189. **Tidskrift i militär helsovård.** Utg. af Svenska militärläkaraföreningen. Stockholm, 1877–1925. T. 1–50. Av. table des tom. 1–30. 50 vol. Av. pl. dont t. 1–39 rel. en 32 vol. d. veau, le reste en livr. 170.—

190. **Transactions, Medico-chirurgical.** London, 1812–14. Vol. 1–5. 5 vols. W. coloured and plain pl. 10.—

191. **Tijdschrift voor genees-, heel-, verlos- en scheikundige wetenschappen.** Uitgeg. d. h. genootschap „Vis Unita Fortior" te Hoorn. Amst. 1824–47. 6 vols. 32.—
All published. 1 Titlepage and 5 indexes missing (if published).

192. **Tijdschrift voor gezondheidsleer.** 's-Grav. 1867–72. 5 vols. 10.—
All published.

193. **Tijdschrift voor ongevallengeneeskunde** (*plus tard*: **Geneeskundig tijdschrift der Rijksverzekeringsbank**). Uitgeg. d. de Rijksverzekeringsbank. Amst. 1916–29. Année 1–14. 14 vol. Av. pl. dont 12 vol. toile, 2 en livr. 40.—
Revue de traitement médical des accidents, publ. par la Banque d'assurance de l'Etat Néerland. contre les accidents.

194. **Tijdschrift ter bevordering der physiolog. genees- en heelkunde.** Breda, 1827–35. 5 vols. 20.—
All published.

195. **Tijdschrift voor staatsgeneeskunde** d. A. Moll. Arnhem, 1843–44. 1 vol. 5.—
All published. Titlepage never published.

196. **Tijdschrift voor wetenschappelijke pharmacie.** 's-Grav. 1849–67. 19 vols. — **Nieuw tijdschrift** voor de pharmacie in Nederland. 's-Grav. 1868–88. Vol. 1–21. — Tog. 40 vols. 100.—
Complete set. It was continued by Nederlansch tijdschrift voor pharmacie.

197. **Tijdschrift, Geneeskundig.** Rott. 1768–71. 4 vols. W. pl. bound. 20.—
All published.

198. **Tijdschrift, Geneeskundig,** voor de zeemacht. 's-Grav. 1863–71. 9 vols. — (*Continued by:*) **Geneeskundig archief** voor de zeemacht. Nieuwediep, 1872–75. 4 vols. — Tog. 13 vols. 50.—
All published.

199. **Tijdschrift, Indisch,** voor geneeskunde. Batavia, 1852–1932. T. 1–71, 72, livr. 1–6. Av. table des tom. 1–65. 74 tom. 68 vol. Av. pl. dont 62 vol. d. rel., le reste en livr. 675.—
La principale revue de médecine des Indes Néerlandaises. Les années

1-5 sont intitulées: Tijdschrift der vereeniging tot bevord. der geneeskundige wetenschappen.
Les exx. complets sont extrêmement rares. Le titre du t. XLI n'existe pas.
Ajouté: **Feestbundel** ter herinnering uitgeg. bij het verschijnen van het
50e deel. Batavia, 1911. Av. ill. toile.

200. **Tijdschrift, Militair-geneeskundig.** Uitgeg. d. J. W. Deknatel, J.
G. Fijan, e.a. Haarlem, 1897-1916. Année 1-20. 20 vol. Av. pl.
et ill. dont 15 vol. cart., 5 en livr.   65.—
Manquent: Année 16, livr. 2 et les titres des années 18-20. Timbres
sur les titres des années 1-15.

201. **Tijdschrift, Nederlandsch,** voor geneeskunde. Orgaan der Nederl. Mij. t. bevord. der geneeskunst. Amst. 1857-1932. Année
1-76. Av. table des années 1857-1906. Année 1-59 rel. en 116 vol.,
année 60-76 en livr.   400.—
La principale revue de médecine néerlandaise; organe de la Société
néerlandaise de médecine.
Ajouté le précurseur: **Tijdschrift** der Nederl. Mij. tot bevordering der
geneeskunst. 's-Grav. 1850-56. 7 vol. rel.

202. **Tijdschrift, Nederlandsch,** voor verloskunde en gynaecologie enz.
Onder red. van H. Treub en G. C. Nijhoff. Haarlem, 1889-1927.
Année 1-31, 32, livr. 1. 31 vol. Av. pl. en couleurs et en noir.
d. rel. unif.   100.—
Série complète de la revue néerlandaise de gynaecologie.

203. **Tijdschrift, Practisch,** voor de geneeskunde in al haren omvang.
Gorinchem, 1821-56. 35 vols. W. 6 suppl. and index to vols.
1-25. Tog. 45 vols. boards.   115.—
All published.

204. **Ugeskrift for Laeger.** Red. af Ahrensen, Kanser, Lehmann, o.a.
Kobenhavn, 1839-1927. Année 1-89. 150 tom. 146 vol. Av. pl.
et figg. dont 19 vol. d. veau, 5 d. rel., 114 cart., le reste en livr.
                                                                         300.—

205. **Unterhaltungsmagazin, Medicinisches und naturwissenschaftli-
ches.** Nordhausen, 1845-47. Vol. 8-10 (last vol. published). 3 vols.
                                                                           2.—
2 Titlepages, 1 index and 2 parts are missing.

206. **Verhandelingen,** bekroond met den prijs van het legaat van J.
Monnikhoff. Amst. 1794-1815. 7 vols. W. pl. Hfcalf.   40.—
All published.

207. **Verhandelingen van het Genootschap ter bevordering der heel-
kunde.** Amst. 1791-1805. 8 vols. — Nieuwe verhandelingen, etc.
Amst. 1808-36. 5 vols. — Prijsverhandelingen. Amst. 1791-1807.
6 vols. — Nieuwe prijsverhandelingen. Amst. 1812-39. 8 vols. —
Tog. 27 vols. W. pl. partly bound.   100.—
All published.

208. **Verhandelingen van het Genootschap Occidit qui non servat.** Antw.,
Dordrecht, 1799-1800. 2 vols.   15.—
All published.

209. **Verhandelingen van de Natuur- en geneeskundige Correspondentie-
societeit.** 's-Grav. 1783-93. 4 vols. in 7. bound.   30.—
All published. 2 indexes are missing.

210. **Verhandelingen en waarnemingen** ter bevorder. der genees-, heel-,
schei- en verloskunde. Leiden, 1801-02. Vol. 1, part 2, 3, vol. 2,
part 1-3.   5.—

211. **Verhandelingen, Genees-, heel-, vroed-, schei- en natuurkundige,** der 1e klasse van het Kon. Nederlandsch Instituut. Amsterdam, 1824–26. 4 vols. W. pl. 4to. 20.—
Reprint of the medical tracts publ. in the vols. 2–7 of the ,,Verhandelingen der 1e klasse van het Kon. Ned. Instituut". Very scarce.

212. **Verhandelingen, Uitgelezene heelkundige,** en waarnemingen, getrokken uit de verzameling van de Haller e. a. werken der beroemste heelkundigen van Europa. Amst., R. Arrenberg, 1759–60. Nos. 1–3. Av. 1 pl. En 1 vol. non rogné. 10.—
Tout ce qui a paru. La plupart des contributions traitent de la maladie des yeux.

213. **Verhandlungen der physikal-medicin. Gesellschaft in Würzburg.** Würzburg, 1850–60. 10 vols. — (*Continued by:*) 1°. **Würzburger medicin. Zeitschrift.** 1860–66. 7 vols.; 2°. **Würzburger naturwisschaftl. Zeitschrift.** 1860-67. 6 vols. — (*Continued by:*) **Verhandlungen der physikal.-medicin. Gesellschaft in Würzburg.** Neue Folge. Würzburg, 1869–75. Vol. 1–8. — Tog. 31 vols. W. pl. bound (1 vol. in parts). 120.—
Complete set. 1 Titlepage missing.

214. **Verslag, Jaarlijksch,** betr. de verpleging en 't onderwijs in het Nederl. gasthuis voor ooglijders (te Utrecht) uitgebr. d. F. C. Donders. M. wetenschapp. bijbladen. Utrecht, 1861–80. Nos. 2–22. En 6 vol. Av. pl. d. veau. *Très rare.* 55.—
Contient plusieurs contributions sur l'ophthalmologie par le prof. F. C. Donders.

215. **Vierteljahrsschrift für gerichtl. und öffentl. Medicin.** Hrsg. von J. L. Casper und H. Eulenberg. Berlin, 1852–80. T. 1–25; Nouv. Série, t. 1–23, 28–33. Av. table des tom. 1–20. 55 tom. 27 vol. Av. pl. d. rel. 65.—
Les pp. 193–200 du t. II manquent.

216. **Vierteljahrsschrift für Psychiatrie.** Neuwied u. Lpz. 1867, 68. 2 vols. W. pl. boards. 7.50
All published.

217. **Watervriend, De,** ter bevordering en uitbreiding der genees- en heelkunst door middel van water. Groningen, 1846–49. Année 1, 3, 4. 3 tom. 1 vol. d. veau. 3.—

218. **Weekblad, Nederlandsch,** voor geneeskundigen. Amst. 1851–56. 6 vols. boards. 15.—
All published.

219. **Werken van het Genootschap ter bevordering der natuur-, genees- en heelkunde te Amsterdam.** Amst. 1871–1926. Série I. 6 vol.; série 2, t. 1–11, 12, nos. 1, 2. Ens. 17 vol., dont 4 br., le reste en livr. 65.—
Travaux de la Société de physiologie et de médecine d'Amsterdam. Le titre et la table des matières du t. 3 de la 2e série n'ont pas paru.

220. **Wochenblatt der Zeitschrift der K. K. Gesellschaft der Aerzte zu Wien.** Wien, 1855–57. Year 1–3. 3 vols. 7.50

221. **Wochenblatt, Medicinisches,** für Aerzte, Wundärzte und Apotheker. Frankfurt, 1780–93. 14 vols. 45.—
All published. 4 Titlepages and indexes missing.

222. **Wochenschrift für die gesammte Heilkunde.** Berlin, 1840–51. Year 8–19. 12 vols. bound. 7.50

223. **Wochenschrift, Oestereichische medicin.,** als Ergänzungsblatt der medicin. Jahrbücher. Wien, 1841–48. 8 vols. 4to and roy. 8vo. boards.   15.—
All published. 5 Titlepages and 5 indexes missing.

224. **Zeitschrift für Diagnostik und Therapie.** Wien, 1882. Year I (all published). boards.   1.50
Titlepage and index missing (if published).

225. **Zeitschrift für practische Heilkunde und Medicinalwesen.** Hannover, 1864–67. 4 vols. boards.   10.—
All published.

226. **Zeitschrift für rationelle Medecin.** Zürich, 1844–69. Series 1, 10 vols; Series 2, 8 vols.; series 3, 36 vols. Tog. 54 vols in 53. boards.   60.—
All published. 2 indexes are missing.

227. **Zeitschrift für die Staatsarzneikunde.** Hrsg. von A. Henke. Erlangen, 1821–64. 88 vols., Ergänz. Hefte 1–29, 36–47 (last publ.) and index to vols. 1–76. Tog. 135 vols. in 104 boards.   75.—
This periodical was discontinued in 1864.

228. **Zeitschrift für Urologie.** Hrsg. von A. Bier, L. Casper u. A. Berlin, 1907–21. T. 1–15. 15 vol.   100.—

229. **Zeitschrift für Veterinärkunde** mit besond. Berücksicht. der Hygiene. Organ für die Veterinäre der Armee. Red. A. Grammlich. Berlin, 1906–16. Année 18–26. 11 vol. Av. figg. dont 8 vol. d. rel., le reste en livr.   20.—

230. **Zeitschrift für wissenschaftliche Therapie.** Berlin, 1853–72. 8 vols. boards.   16.—
All published.

231. **Zeitschrift, Gemeinsame deutsche,** für Geburtskunde. Weimar, 1826–32. Vol. 1, 4–7. 5 vols. — (*Continued by*:) **Neue gemeinsame deutsche Zeitschrift für Geburtskunde.** Berlin, 1840–52. Vol. 9–33. 24 vols. — (*Continued by*:) **Monatsschrift für Geburtskunde und Frauenkrankheiten.** Berlin, 1852–69. Vol. 1–34 (last vol. publ.). In 35 vols. — Tog. 64 vols. W. pl. boards.   65.—
1 Index missing.

232. **Zeitschrift, Schweizerische,** für Heilkunde. Bern, 1862–64. 3 vols. boards.   10.—
All published.

233. **Zeitschrift, Schweizerische,** für Medicin, Chirurgie und Geburtshülfe. Hrsg. von der medizin-chirurg. Kantonalgesellschaften von Zürich und Bern. Bern, Zürich, 1842–52. Année 1–11. 11 vol. Av. pl. cart.   30.—
La table de l'année 1851 manque.

234. **Zeitung, Medicinisch-chirurgische.** Innsbruck, 1790–1810, 1828–32, 1838–56 (last year publ.). 165 vols. in 138, of which 102 vols. bound.   75.—
Set from the commencement. 6 titlepages and 2 indexes are missing.

235. **Zeitung, Medizinische.** Berlin, 1832–37. Year 1–6. 3 vols. fol. hfcalf.   7.50

236. **Zentralblatt für die gesamte Chirurgie und ihre Grenzgebiete.** Hrsg. von A. Bier u. A. Berlin, 1913–20. T. 1–6. 6 vol. En livr.   20.—

Prices are in Dutch guilders

237. **Zentralblatt für die gesamte Gynaekologie und Geburtshilfe** sowie deren Grenzgebiete. Hrsg. von O. Beuttner, A. Doderlein, B. Krönig u. A. Berlin, 1913–14. T. 1–3. 3 vol. En livr.   12.—

MEDICAL CONGRESSES

INTERNATIONAL

238. **Congrès internat. médical** des accidents du travail. Liége 1905. Rapports et communications. Compte rendu des séances.   10.—

239. **Congrès internat.**, 7e, des accidents et des maladies du travail. Bruxelles 1935. Rapports. 3 vols.   8.—

240. — 8e, des accoucheuses. Paris 1938. Compte rendu.   1.25

241. — 2e, de l'alimentation. Liége 1911. Rapports. 2 vols.   7.—

242. **Congrès scientifique internat.**, 2e, de l'alimentation. Paris 1937. La science de l'alimentation en 1937. Compte rendu des séances et discussions des rapports.   3.—

243. **Congrès internat.** pour l'amélioration du sort des aveugles. Paris 1900. (Compte rendu des séances. Mémoires).   4.—

244. **Congrès universel** pour l'amélioration du sort des aveugles et des sourds-muets. Paris 1878. Comptes rendus sténograph.   6.—

245. **Kongresz, 4er Internat. Anatomen-.** Mailand 1936. Verhandlungen der Anatomischen Gesellschaft. W. 2 pl. and 95 figg.   9.50
    Ergänz. Heft z. 83. Bd. des Anatomischen Anzeigers.

246. **Congressus internat.**, 5., medicorum pro artificibus calamitate afflictis aegrotisque. Budapest 1928. Opera collecta.   16.—
    Although the title is in latin, the articles are in english, french or german.

247. **Kongress, 3er Internat.**, für das ärztliche Fortbildungswesen. (Medical postgraduate study). Berlin 1937. Bericht. bound.   15.—

248. **Congrès internat.** de l'assistance des aliénés et spécialement de leur assistance familiale. Anvers 1902. Rapports et compte-rendu des séances.   10.—

249. — 1er, de l'asthme. Le Mont Dore 1932. Rapports. Communications et discussions.   5.50

250. — des auxiliaires médicaux et 1er Congrès internat. de massage. Paris 1937. [Compte rendu]. 4to.   3.—

251. **Conférence internat.**, 1re, de bains populaires et scolaires. Schéveningue 1912. Compte-rendu des travaux. bound.   4.—

252. **Kongress** zur Bekämpfung der Tuberkulose als Volkskrankheit. Berlin 1899. Bericht. bound.   3.50

252a. **Conférence internat.**, 2e, pour l'étude du cancer. Paris 1910. Travaux.   8.—

253. **Congrès** de la Société internat. de chirurgie. Bruxelles 1905. Procès-verbaux, rapports et discussions. bound.   10.—

254. — 2e, de la Société internat. de chirurgie. Bruxelles 1908. Procès-verbaux, discussions, rapports. 2 vols. bound.   12.—

255. — 3e, de la Société internat. de chirurgie. Bruxelles 1911. Rapports, procès-verbaux et discussions. bound.   8.—

256. — 4e, de la Société internat. de chirurgie. New York 1914. Rapports, procès-verbaux et discussions. W. pl. bound.   8.50

257. **Congrès,** 5e, de la Société internat. de chirurgie. Paris 1920. Rapports, procès-verbaux et discussions. W. pl. bound.   8.50
258. — 9e, de la Société internat. de chirurgie. Madrid 1932. Rapports, procès-verbaux et discussions. 3 vols.   20.—
259. — 10e, de la Société internat. de chirurgie. Le Caire 1935, 36. Rapports, procès-verbaux et discussions. 3 vols. bound.   20.—
260. — 1er, de la Société internat. de chirurgie orthopédique. Paris 1930. Procès-verbaux, rapports et discussions. bound.   7.50
261. — 2e, de la Société internat. de chirurgie orthopédique. Londres 1933. Procès-verbaux, rapports, discussions et communic. particul. bound. (650 pp.).   20.—
262. **Congrès européen, 1er,** de chirurgie structive. Bruxelles 1936. [Compte rendu]. In parts.   8.—
      Printed in Revue de chirurgie structive, 1936, nos. 3 et 4 and 1937, no. 1.
263. **Congress, 3d World,** of the Internat. Society for crippled children. Budapest 1936. Proceedings.   10.—
264. **Conférence (internat.)** de la défense sociale contre le syphilis. Nancy 1928. Rapports. Procès-verbaux. 2 vols.   9.—
265. **Centenaire d'Alfred Fournier.** Conférence internat. de défense sociale contre le syphilis. Paris 1932. Rapports. Compte rendu. 2 vols.   9.50
266. **Congrès dentaire interalliés.** Paris 1916. Comptes rendus. 2 vols. W. 1100 figg.   20.—
267. — **dentaire internat.,** 8e, Paris 1931. Compte rendu général, rapports généraux et conférence. 4to.   35.—
268. **Congress, 6th Internat. dental.** London 1914. Transactions. bound.   6.—
269. — **7th Internat. dental.** Philadelphia 1926. Transactions. 2 vols. bound.   15.—
      For the greater part reprinted from the Journal of the American dental Association.
270. **Kongress, 5er Internat. Dermatologen-.** Berlin 1904. Verhandlungen und Berichte. 3 vols. in 2. bound.   12.—
271. **Congress, 6th Internat. dermatological.** New York 1907. Offic. transactions. 2 vols. W. pl. bound.   12.—
272. **Congrès internat.** de dermatologie et de syphiligraphie. Paris 1889. Comptes rendus. bound.   10.—
273. **Congrès, 1er,** des dermatologistes et syphiligraphes de langue française. Paris 1922. (Rapports).   5.—
274. — 4e, des dermatologistes et syphiligraphes de langue française. Paris 1929. Rapport. Discussions et communications. 2 vols.   8.—
275. — 5e, des dermatologistes et syphiligraphes de langue française. Lyon 1934. Rapports.   7.50
276. **Congressus dermatologorum internat. IX.** Budapest 1935. Deliberationes. 5 vols. in 7. W. pl. and figg.   210.—
      Contains contributions in english, french, german and italian. Vol. V, comprising 3 vols., contains an atlas of 4566 figg.
277. — Idem. Vol. V. Corpus iconum morborum cutaneorum. Coll. et ed. L. Nekam. 1 vol. text and 2 vols. w. 4566 ill. Tog. 3 vols.   135.—
278. **Congrès** pour favoriser le développement des stations hydro-

Prices are in Dutch guilders

minérales maritimes, climatiques et alpines des nations alliées. Monaco 1920. Congrès de l'alpinisme. Comptes rendus. 2 vols. 7.50

279. **Congrès internat.**, 1er, d'électrologie et de radiologie médicales. Paris 1900. W. 9 pl. 10.—

280. — 2e, d'électrologie et de radiologie médicales. Berne 1902. Comptes-rendus des séances. 8.50

281. — 5e, d'électrologie et de radiologie médicales. Barcelone 1910. [Comptes rendus]. vellum. 10.—

282. **Congresso internaz.**, 1ro, di elettro-radio-biologia. Venezia 1934. Atti. 2 vols. W. pl. and figg. bound. 24.—
    Archivio internaz. di radiobiologia generale. Vol. II, III.

283. **Conference, 1st Internat.**, of fever therapy. New York 1937. 14.—

284. **Congresso internaz.**, 14ᵉ, di fisiologia. Roma 1932. Conferenze e sunti delle comunicazioni. 10.—
    Archivio di scienze biologiche. Vol. XVIII, nos. 1-4.

285. **Congrès internat.**, 1er, de gastro-entérologie. Bruxelles 1935. Procès-verbaux, rapports et discussions. bound. 15.—

286. — Idem. Informations et Rapports. 7.50

287. — 2e, de gastro-entérologie. Paris 1937. Procès-verbaux, etc. bound. 15.—

288. **Kongress, 6er Internat.**, für Geburtshülfe und Gynäkologie. Berlin 1912. Verhandlungen. 6.—

289. — 1er Internat., für gerichtliche und soziale Medizin. Bonn 1938. Verhandlungsbericht. 18.50

290. **Conférence internat.**, 2e, du goître. Berne 1933. Compte rendu. 12.—

291. **Congrès internat.**, 1er, des gouttes de lait. Paris 1905. Rapports. Communications. Discussion. 5.—

292. — 2e, des gouttes de lait. Protection de l'enfance du premier âge. Bruxelles 1907. Compte rendu. 3.50

293. — de gymnastique pédagogique, militaire, médicale et esthétique. Bruxelles 1910. Rapport général. 4.—

294. **Congrès périodique internat.**, 1er, de gynécologie et d'obstétrique. Bruxelles 1892. Compte rendu. 7.50

295. — 2e, de gynécologie et d'obstétrique. Genève 1896. Comptes-rendus. 3 vols. 12.—

296. — 3e, de gynécologie et d'obstétrique. Amsterdam 1899. Compte-rendu. 8.—

297. — 4e, de gynécologie et d'obstétrique. Rome 1902. Comptes-rendus. 6.50

298. **Congrès**, 2e, (de l')Association des gynécologues et obstétriciens de langue française. Paris 1921. Rapports. Discussion des rapports et communications. 2 vols. 5.—
    Publ. in „Revue gynécologique et obstétrique".

299. — 3e, (de l')Association des gynécologues et obstétriciens de langue française. Paris 1923. Rapports, discussions et communications. 2.50
    Publ. in „Revue gynécologique et obstétrique".

300. — 6e, (de l')Association des gynécologues et obstétriciens de langue française. Bruxelles 1929. Rapports, discussions et communications. 3.50
    Publ. in „Revue gynécologique et obstétrique".

301. **Congrès internat.**, 8e, de haute culture médicale. Athènes 1936.
Compte rendu.   8.—
302. **Congrès national et internat.**, 1er, de l'herboristerie, de la pro-
duction et du commerce des plantes médicinales. Paris 1937.
Communications et rapports.   4.50
303. **Congrès internat.**, 1er, de l'histoire de l'art de guérir. Anvers 1920.
Liber memorialis.   5.—
304. — 2e, d'histoire de la médecine. Paris 1921. Compte rendu.   9.—
305. —, 3e, d'histoire des sciences. Portugal 1934. Actes, confé-
rences et communications. W. portraits, large maps and pl. 4to.
(463 pp.).   15.—
   Contains a.o.: **Ricardo Jorge, A.,** La médecine et les médecins dans
   l'expansion mondiale des Portugais. — **F. da Costa,** La science nautique
   des Portugais à l'époque des découvertes. — **Q. Vetter,** Relations mathé-
   matiques entre les pays Tchèques et les pays de la Péninsule Ibérique,
   l'Amérique et l'Extrême Orient. — **A. Camilo Monteiro,** De l'influence
   portugaise au Japon. — **M. Meyerhof,** Esquisse d'histoire de la pharma-
   cologie et de la botanique chez les Musulmans d'Espagne. — **H. P. J.
   Renaud,** Introd. des drogues végétales américaines dans la matière médicale des arabes. — **F. Jaguaribe de Mattos,** Les idées sur la physiographie
   sud-américaine. — etc.
306. — d'homœpathie. Paris 1878. Comptes rendus sténograph.   5.—
307. — d'homœopathie. Paris 1900. Compte rendu.   12.—
308. — 1er, des hopitaux. Atlantic city 1929. [Rapports et discus-
sions].   4.—
309. — 4e, d'hydrologie, de climatologie et de géologie. Clermont-
Ferrand 1896. Compte-rendu. bound.   9.—
310. — 5e, d'hydrologie, de climatologie et de géologie. Liége, 1898.
bound.   7.50
311. — 6e, d'hydrologie, de climatologie et de géologie. Grenoble
1902. Compte rendu. bound.   7.50
312. — 12e, d'hydrologie, de climatologie et de géologie médicales.
Lyon 1927. Rapports. Communications. 2 vols. *Rare.*   15.—
313. — 15e, d'hydrologie, de climatologie et de géologie médicales.
Belgrado 1936. Rapports.   12.—
314. — d'hygiène. Paris 1878. Comptes rendus sténograph. 2 vol. 12.50
315. — 5e, d'hygiène et de démographie. La Haye 1884. Comptes
rendus et mémoires.   9.—
316. — d'hygiène et de démographie. Paris 1889. Compte rendu.
bound. (1267 pp.).   8.—
317. — 8e, d'hygiène et de démographie. Budapest 1894. Comptes-
rendus et mémoires. Vol. I, III, IV. 3 vols.   Each vol. 2.—
318. — 10e, d'hygiène et de démographie. Paris 1900. Compte rendu.
(1070 pp.).   9.—
319. — 13e, d'hygiène et de démographie. Bruxelles 1903. Compte-
rendu. 9 vols. of which 8 bound.   40.—
320. **Kongress, 14er Internat.,** für Hygiene und Demographie. Berlin
1907. Bericht. 4 vols in 5.   25.—
   Added: **Kongressblatt.** 23 et 24 sept. 1907. Nos. 1, 2. — **Medizin. An-
   stalten** a. d. Gebiete der Volksgesundheitspflege in Preuszen. — **M. Kirch-
   ner,** Die gesetzl. Grundlagen der Seuchenbekämpfung im Deutschen
   Reiche, bes. Preuszens. — **Besuch** in Hamburg. Jena, Hamburg, 1907.
   3 vols.

Prices are in Dutch guilders

321. **Congrès internat.** d'hygiène, de sauvetage et d'économie sociale. Bruxelles 1876. 2 vols. bound.   12.—
322. — d'hygiène méditerranéenne. Marseille 1932. Rapports et comptes rendus. 2 vols. bound.   15.—
323. — 2e, d'hygiène mentale. Paris 1937. Comptes rendus.   12.50
324. — 3e, d'hygiène scolaire. Paris 1910. Rapports. Résumé de rapports et de communications. Compte rendu. 3 vols.   13.50
325. **Congrès interallié** d'hygiène sociale pour la reconstitution des régions dévastées par la guerre. Paris 1919. Compte rendu général des travaux. 4 vols.   18.—
326. **Congrès internat.** de propagande d'hygiène sociale et d'éducation prophylactique sanitaire et morale. Paris 1923. Rapports.   5.50
327. — 2e, de l'hypnotisme expérimental et thérapeutique. Paris 1900. Comptes rendus.   5.—
328. **Congrès internat.** de l'insuffisance hépatique. Vichy 1937. Rapports. Comptes rendus, discussions et communications diverses. 2 vols. (1365 pp.).   20.—
329. **Kongress, 4er Internat.,** für Kinderheilkunde. Rom 1937. Verhandlungen.   12.—
      Acta paediatrica. Bd XXII.
330. — **Internat.,** für Kurzwellen in Physik, Biologie und Medizin. Wien 1937. Referate und Mitteilungen.   5.50
331. — **1er Internat. Laryngo-Rhinologen-.** Wien 1908. Verhandlungen. (12.—)   7.50
332. — **3er Internat. Laryngo-Rhinologen-.** Berlin 1911. Tl II. Verhandlungen.   3.50
333. — **3er Internat.,** für Lichtforschung. Wiesbaden 1936. Kongressbericht. bound.   25.—
      Very important medical congress.
334. **Congress, 1st Internat.,** on life assurance medicine. London 1935. Transactions.   10.—
335. **Congrès internat.** de la lithiase biliaire. Vichy 1932. 2 vols.   7.50
336. **Kongress, 5er,** der Internat. Gesellschaft für Logopädie und Phoniatrie. Wien 1932. Bericht über die Verhandlungen.   9.—
337. — 6er, der Internat. Gesellschaft für Logopädie und Phoniatrie. Budapest 1934. Bericht über die Verhandlungen.   6.—
      Partly published in Monatsschrift für Ohrenheilkunde und Laryngo-Rhinologie.
338. **Congrès internat.,** 2e, de la lumière. Biologie, biophysique, thérapeutique. bound.   15.—
339. — 2e, de lutte scientifique et sociale contre le cancer. Bruxelles 1936. Travaux scientifiques. 3 vols. 4to. (25.—)   20.—
340. — du lymphatisme. La Bourboule 1934. Rapports. Comptes rendus et communications.   5.—
341. — 2e, des maladies professionnelles. Bruxelles 1910. Actes. Rapports et communications.   7.50
342. — 12e, de médecine. Moscou 1897. Comptes-rendus. 7 vols. in 8.   30.—
343. — 13e, de médecine. Paris 1900. Section de chirurgie générale. Comptes rendus.   5.—
      Added: Idem. Organisation. Assemblées générales.

Mart. Nijhoff, The Hague — Cat. No. 629

Prices are in Dutch guilders

367. **Congrès internat.,** 8e, de médecine vétérinaire. Budapest 1905. Compte rendu. 3 vols. in 1. bound. 12.—
368. — 11e, de médecine vétérinaire (veterinary). Londres 1930. Compte rendu. 3 vols. in 1. hfbound. 12.—
369. **Congrès,** 13e, des médecins aliénistes et neurologistes de France et des pays de langue française. Bruxelles 1903. 2 vols. 7.50
370. — 20e, des médecins aliénistes et neurologistes de France et des pays de langue française. Bruxelles-Liége 1910. Vol. I. Rapports. 2.50
371. — 28e, des médecins aliénistes et neurologistes de France et des pays de langue française. Bruxelles 1921. Comptes rendus. 4.50
372. — 37e, des médecins aliénistes et neurologistes de France et des pays de langue française. Rabat 1933. Comptes rendus. 6.50
373. — 38e, des médecins aliénistes et neurologistes de France et des pays de langue française. Lyon 1934. Comptes rendus. 6.50
374. **Congrès internat.,** 1er, des médecins de compagnies d'assurances. Bruxelles 1899. Rapports, procès-verbaux des séances. 3.50
375. — 2e, des médecins de compagnies d'assurances. Amsterdam 1901. Rapports, procès-verbaux des séances. 7.50
376. — 3e, des médecins de compagnies d'assurances. Paris 1903. Rapports. Procès-verbaux des séances. 2 vols. 5.—
377. **Congress, 7th Internat. medical.** London 1881. Transactions. 4 vols. W. pl. and ill. bound. 20.—
    Added: Abstracts of the communications to be made in the various sections. 1881. bound.
378. **Congresso internaz.** della medicina dello sport. Torino, Roma 1933. Atti. 4.50
379. **Congresso** della Lega internaz. di medicina omiopatica. Roma 1930. Atti. W. pl. 13.50
380. **Congress, 10er Internat. medicinischer.** Berlin 1890. Verhandlungen. 5 vols. 15.—
381. **Congreso medico centroamericano,** 2°. San Jose 1934. Memorias. San Jose, Costarica, 1935. W. portr. and pl. 9.—
382. **Congresso medico internaz.,** 11°. Roma 1894. Atti. 6 vols. 20.—
383. **Woche, 1e Internat. medizinische,** in der Schweiz. Montreux 1935. Vorträge. 10.—
384. — **2e Internat. medizinische,** in der Schweiz. Luzern 1936. 10.—
385. **Kongress, 1er Internat. Neurologen-.** Bern 1931. Bericht. 7.50
386. **Conferencia,** 1ra, latino-americana de neurologia, psiquiatria y medicina legal. Buenos Aires 1928. Actas. 2 vols. 20.—
387. **Congrès internat.,** 1er, de neurologie, de psychiatrie, d'électricité médicale et d'hyppologie. Bruxelles 1897. Rapports, Communications, Résumés. 3 vols. 6.—
388. **Congress, 7th,** of Scandinavian neurologists. Oslo 1936. Report. 5.—
    Acta psychiatrica et neurologica. Vol. XII, fasc. 4.
389. **Congres, 4e Internat.,** voor ongevallengeneeskunde en beroepsziekten. Amsterdam 1925. Handelingen. bound. 5.—
390. **Congress, 7er Internat. Ophtalmologen-.** Heidelberg 1888. W. 8 pl. and figg. bound. 15.—

391. **Concilium ophthalmologicum, 13.** Amsterdam–Den Haag 1929. 5 vols. W. numer. pl. and ill. bound. (1 vol. sewed). 48.—
I–II. Compte-rendu. — III. Symposia. — IV. Rapports. — V. Résumés.
392. **Congrès internat.**, 2e, d'ophthalmologie. Paris 1862. Compte-rendu. bound. 14.—
393. — 9e, d'ophthalmologie. Utrecht 1899. Compte rendu. W. pl. bound. 14.—
394. — 10e, d'ophthalmologie. Lucerne 1904. Compte-rendu. W. pl. bound. 8.—
395. — 3e, d'otologie. Bâle 1884. Comptes-rendus et mémoires. 5.—
396. — 4e, d'otologie. Bruxelles 1888. Comptes-rendus et Mémoires. bound. 7.50
397. — 5e, d'otologie. Florence 1895. Comptes-rendus et Mémoires. 5.—
398. — 7e, d'otologie. Bordeaux 1904. Compte rendu. 7.50
399. — 10e, d'otologie. Paris 1922. Rapports. Comptes rendus des séances. 2 vols. 8.50
400. **Kongress, 3er Internat. Oto-Rhino-Laryngologen-.** Berlin 1936. Verhandlungen. 2 vols. 35.—
Zeitschrift f. Hals-, Nasen- u. Ohrenheilkunde. Bd 40, H. 1–5.
401. **Congrès**, 1er, de la Societas oto-rhino-laryngologica Latina. Madrid 1929. Rapports. Compte rendu, etc. 2 vols. 10.—
402. — 2e, de la Societas, oto-rhino-laryngologica Latina. Catane 1931. Rapports. Compte rendu, etc. 2 vols. 10.—
403. — 3e, de la Societas oto-rhino-laryngologica Latina. Paris 1933. Rapports. Compte rendu, etc. 2 vols. 10.—
404. — 4e, de la Societas oto-rhino-laryngologica Latina. Bruxelles 1935. Relationes. Acta. 10.—
405. **Congrès internat.**, 1er, du paludisme. Rome 1925. Compte-rendu. 4to. 20.—
406. **Congress, 6th Scandinavian pathological.** Oslo 1935. Transactions. 5.—
Acta pathologica et microbiologica Scandinavia. Suppl. XXVI.
406a. **Congrès internat.**, 1er, de pathologie comparée. Paris 1912. Rapports. Comptes rendus et communications. 2 vols. in 3. 12.—
407. — 2e, de pathologie comparée. 1931. Rapports, Comptes rendus et communications. 2 vols. 7.50
408. — 3e, de pathologie comparée. Athènes 1936. Rapports. Comptes rendus et communications. 4 vols. 18.50
409. **Conférence internat.**, 2e, de pathologie géographique. Utrecht 1934. Comptes rendus. 7.50
410. — Idem. Résumé des rapports, Programme, etc. 1.50
411. **Congress, 7th Northern pediatric.** Oslo 1938. Proceedings. 6.—
Acta paediatrica. Vol. XXIV.
412. **Congrès internat.**, 2e, de pédiatrie. Stockholm 1930. 5.—
Publ. in „Acta paediatrica".
413. — 3e, de pédiatrie. London 1933. 10.—
Publ. in „Acta paediatrica".
414. **Conférence**, 1re–4e, (de l')Association Internat. de pédiatrie préventive. La Haye 1931, Genève 1932, Luxembourg 1933, Lyon 1934. Comptes rendus. 4 vols. 6.50

Prices are in Dutch guilders

415. **Congrès internat.,** 1er, de pédologie. Bruxelles 1911. Comptes rendus. Rapports. 2 vols. 12.—
416. — 6e, pharmaceutique. Bruxelles 1885. Compte rendu. bound. (C + 905 + 242 pp.). 12.—
417. — 8e, de pharmacie. Bruxelles 1897. Compte rendu. 5.—
418. — 9e, de pharmacie. Paris 1900. Compte rendu. bound. 7.50
419. — 10e, de pharmacie. Bruxelles 1910. Compte rendu. 5.—
420. — 11e, de pharmacie. La Haye-Schéveningue 1913. Compte-rendu. 2 vols. 10.—
421. — 12e, de pharmacie. Bruxelles 1935. Comptes rendus. Rapports. 7.50
421a. **Congress,** 1st Internat., of phonetic sciences. Amsterdam 1932. Proceedings. 6.—
   Archives néerland. de phonétique expérimentale. T. VIII, IX.
421b. — **3d Internat.,** of phonetic sciences. Ghent 1938. Proceedings. 9.—
422. **Congrès internat.** de phréniatrie et de neuropathologie. Anvers 1885. [Rapports]. Mémoires divers. Compte rendu. 5.—
423. **Kongress, 16er Internat. Physiologen-.** Zürich 1938. Kongressbericht. 3 vols. 6.50
424. **Congress, 15th Internat. physiological.** Leningrad-Moscow 1935. Proceedings. 9.—
   The Sechenov journal of physiology. Vol. XXI, nr. 5-6.
425. **Congrès internat.,** 1er, physiothérapie. Liége 1905. Compte-rendu des séances. 4.—
426. — 3e, de physiothérapie. Rapports. Comptes rendus et communications. 2 vols. 7.50
427. **Congrès,** 1er, de physiothérapie des médecins de langue française. Paris 1908. Compte rendu des travaux. 3.—
428. — 3e, de physiothérapie des médecins de langue française. Paris 1911. Vol. II. Comptes-rendus des séances. 1.50
429. **Conference, Internat. plague.** Mukden 1911. Report. bound. 10.—
430. **Congresso internaz.,** 5°, di psicologia. Roma 1905. Atti. 7.50
431. **Congrès internat.,** 1er, de psychiatrie, de neurologie, de psychologie et de l'assistance des aliénés. Amsterdam 1907. Compte rendu des travaux. 2 vols. 10.—
432. — 1er, de psychiatrie infantile. Paris 1937. Rapports. Comptes rendus. 4 vols. 12.50
433. **Congress, 4th Internat.,** for psychical research. Athens 1930. Transactions. 4.—
434. — **3er Internat.,** für Psychologie. München 1896. [Verhandlungen]. 6.—
435. **Congrès internat.,** 4e, de psychologie. Paris 1900. Compte rendu des séances et textes des mémoires. 7.50
436. — 6e, de psychologie. Genève 1909. Rapports et comptes-rendus. 10.—
437. — 11e, de psychologie. Paris 1937. Rapports et comptes rendus. W. 25 pl. bound. 9.—
438. — 2e, de psychologie expérimentale. Paris 1913. Compte rendu des travaux. 6.50

439. **Congress, 10th Internat.**, of psychology. Copenhagen 1932. Papers.
8.—
Acta psychologica. Ed. a G. Révész. I, 1.
440. **Conférence internat.**, 4e, de psychotechnique. Paris 1927. Comptes rendus.   7.50
441. — 5e, de psychotechnique. Utrecht 1928. Comptes rendus. 6.—
442. — 8e, de psychotechnique. Prague 1934. Compte rendu. 13.50
443. **Congrès internat.**, 4e, de radiesthésie. Paris 1935. Compte rendu.
4.—
Bull. de l'Assoc. des amis de la radiesthésie. No. 33 (No. spécial).
444. **Kongress, 4er Internat. Radiologen-.** Zürich 1934. 4 vols. W. hundreds of portr. and pl. bound.   25.—
I. Teilnehmerverzeichnisz und Porträtkatalog. — II. Referate. — III. Organisation der Krebsbekämpfung. — IV. Schluszbericht.
445. **Congrès internat.**, 3e, de radiologie. Paris 1931. Rapports et communications. bound.   13.50
446. — Idem. Résumés des communications.   3.50
447. **Congress, 2d Internat.**, of radiology. Stockholm 1928. Abstracts of communications.   1.—
448. **Conférence internat.**, 1re, du rat. Paris–Le Havre 1928. Documents.   8.—
449. — 2e, et congrès colonial du rat et de la peste. Paris 1931. Documents. W. 86 figg.   8.50
450. **Congrès internat.**, 1er, des recherches psychiques. Copenhague 1921. Compte rendu offic. boards.   8.—
451. — 2e, des recherches psychiques. (Psychical research). Varsovie 1923. [Compte rendu].   3.—
The compte rendu bears the following title: L'état actuel des recherches psychiques d'après les travaux du congrès.
452. — 3e, de recherches psychiques. (Psychical research). Paris 1927. Compte rendu.   5.—
453. — 1er, pour la répression des fraudes alimentaires et pharmaceutiques. Genève 1908. Compte rendu des travaux.   7.50
454. — 2e, pour la répression des fraudes concern. les denrées alimentaires, les matières premières de la droguerie, les huiles essentielles, etc. Paris 1909. Compte rendu.   12.50
455. **Conférence** pour la répression du trafic illicite des drogues nuisibles. Genève 1936. Comptes rendus des débats. 4to.   4.50
Série de publ. de la Société des Nations. 11, 1936, 20.
456. **Congrès internat.**, 3e, de rhumatisme. Paris 1932. Rapports et communications.   5.—
457. **Conférence scientifique internat.** du rhumatisme chronique progressif généralisé. Aix-les-Bains 1934. 2 vols.   12.—
458. **Conferencia sanitaria internac.**, 5a, de las Repúblicas Americanas. Santiago de Chile 1911.   8.—
459. **Conference, Internat.**, on sanitary engineering. London 1924. Transactions. bound.   4.—
460. **Kongress, 3er Internat.**, für Säuglingsschutz (gouttes de lait). Berlin 1911. Bericht. (1256 pp.).   12.—
461. — Idem. Säuglingsfürsorge in Grosz-Berlin. bound.   4.—

Prices are in Dutch guilders

462. **Congrès internat.**, 3e, de sauvetage et de premiers secours en cas d'accidents. (Reddingwezen en eerste hulp bij ongelukken). Amsterdam 1926. Compte rendu. 10.—
463. — 4e, de sauvetage et de premiers secours en cas d'accidents. (Redningskongres). København 1934. 12.—
464. **Congrès périodique internat.**, 5e, des sciences médicales. Genève 1877. Comptes-rendus et mémoires. 6.—
465. — 6e, des sciences médicales. Amsterdam 1879. Compte rendu. 2 vols. 7.50
466. **Congrès internat.** sur le service médical des armées en campagne. Paris 1878. Comptes rendus sténograph. 4.—
467. **Congress, 2d Sexual reform.** Copenhagen 1928. Proceedings. 7.50
468. **Kongress,** 4er, für Sexualreform. Wien 1930. Sexualnot und Sexualreform. Verhandlungen der Weltliga für Sexualreform. W. 6 pl. 20.—
469. **Conférence internat.** (de) la silicose. Johannesburg 1930. Compte rendu. (741 pp.). 7.50
Bureau Internat. du travail. Etudes et documents. Série F. (Hygiène industrielle). No. 13.
470. **Congrès internat.**, 2d, des sourds-muets. Chicago 1893. [Rapports]. 4.—
471. **Kongress, 2er Internat. Sportärzte-.** Berlin 1936. Verhandlungsbericht. W. 115 ill. 16.—
472. **Congrès internat.**, 1er, des stations balnéaires. Budapest 1937. Compte rendu des travaux. 18.50
473. **Congresso internaz.**, 2°, di stomatologia. Bologna 1935. Atti. 2 vols. 25.—
474. **Congrès stomatologique internat.**, 1er. Budapest 1931. Compte rendu. 2 vols. bound. 15.—
475. **Congresso internaz.**, 8°, di storia della medicina. Roma 1930. Atti. 13.50
476. **Kongress** für synthetische Lebensforschung. Marienbad 1936. Verhandlungsbericht über die Aussprache zw. Ärzten, Biologen, etc. 4.50
477. **Conférence (internat.)** de la syphilis héréditaire. Paris 1925. Rapports. Procès-verbaux. 2 vols. 9.—
478. **Congrès internat.**, 3e, de technique sanitaire et d'hygiène urbaine. Lyon 1932. Comptes rendus et communications. 4to. 12.—
479. **Congresso internaz.**, 2°, di terapia fisica. Roma 1907. Atti. Vol. I. W. 4 pl. 6.—
480. **Congrès**, 1er, de l'Association internat. de thalasssothérapie. Cannes 1914. Rapports. Comptes-rendus des séances. 2 vols. 15.—
481. **Congrès internat.**, 6e, de thalassothérapie. Berek 1931. 3.—
482. **Kongress, 1er Internat.**, der Therapeutischen Union. Bern 1937. Verhandlungsbericht. 11.50
483. **Congrès internat.** du tourisme, du thermalisme et du climatisme. Paris 1937. Rapports. 4to. In 21 parts. 10.—
Official dactylographed and polycopied publication. Each part forms a whole section.

Mart. Nijhoff, The Hague — Cat. No. 629

484. **Congress,** 9th, (of the) Far Eastern Association of tropical medicine. Nanking 1934. [Transactions and Proceedings]. 2 vols.   25.—
485. **Congrès internat.** de la tuberculose. Paris 1905. 5 vols.   24.—
486. **Conférence,** 8e, de l'Union internat. contre la tuberculose. La Haye–Amsterdam 1932. Rapports.   9.—
487. **Congrès (internat.),** 2e, pour l'étude de la tuberculose chez l'homme et chez les animaux. Paris 1891. Comptes rendus et mémoires.   7.50
488. — 3e, pour l'étude de la tuberculose chez l'homme et chez les animaux. Paris 1893. Comptes rendus et mémoires.   6.—
489. — 4e, pour l'étude de la tuberculose chez l'homme et chez les animaux. Paris 1898. Comptes rendus et mémoires.   7.50
490. **Congress, 6th Internat.,** on tuberculosis. Washington 1908. Proceedings. Report, etc. Public lectures. 6 vols in 8.   40.—
491. **Kongress, 8er Internat.,** für Unfallmedizin und Berufskrankheiten. Frankfurt a.M. 1938. Bericht. 2 vols. W. 145 ill.   28.50
492. **Congress,** 4°, de la Sociedad internac. de urologia. Madrid 1930. Ponencias offic. Discusion. 2 vols.   8.—
493. **Kongress,** 6er, der Internat. Gesellschaft für Urologie. Wien 1936. Referate. Diskussionen. 2 vols.   10.—
493. **Congress,** 5th, of the Internat. Society of urology. London 1933. Reports. Discussions.   8.—
495. **Congres, Internat.,** voor verloskunde en gynaecologie. Amsterdam 1938. Handelingen. (Report of the activities). 2 vols.   20.—
496. **Kongress, 4er Internat.,** für Versicherungs-Medizin. Berlin 1906. Berichte und Verhandlungen. bound.   7.50
497. **Kongress, 3er Veterinaer-,** der Baltischen Staaten. Kaunas 1937. Referate. Protokolle. 2 vols.   4.50
498. **Convegni Volta,** 1°–4°. Roma 1931–1934. Atti. 5 vols.   20.—
   1°, 1931. Tema: La fisica nucleare. 2.25 — 2°, 1932. Tema: L'Europa. 2 vols. 7.75. — 3°, 1933. Tema: L'immunologia. 7.75. — 4°, 1934. Tema: Teatro. 2.25.
499. **Kongresz, 9er Internat. Zahnärzte-.** Wien 1936. Berichte. Vol. I. W. ill. (1552 pp.).   20.—
500. **Kongress, 5er Internat. zahnärztlicher.** Berlin 1909. Verhandlungen. 2 vols. W. pl. bound.   12.50

NATIONAL

501. **Réunion,** 28e, de l'Association des Anatomistes et 1re de la Société Anatomique Portugaise. Lisbonne 1933. Comptes rendus. (711 pp.).   15.—
   Bulletin de l'Association des Anatomistes. No. 32.
502. **Congrès** de l'arthritisme. Vittel 1927.   2.—
   Revue médicale de l'Est, 1927, no. 21bis.
503. — 1er, de la Ligue (nationale belge contre le cancer). Bruxelles 1923. Rapports.   2.—
504. **Congress,** 28er–46er, der deutschen Gesellschaft für Chirurgie. 1899–1922. Verhandlungen. 19 vols. W. pl. bound (except 3).   90.—
   Added: **Verhandlungen** des 50. Congresses. 1926.
505. **Tagung,** 61e, der deutschen Gesellschaft für Chirurgie. Be lin, 1937. W. 3 pl. and 275 figgs.   27.50
   Archiv f. klinische Chirurgie. Bd 189.

Prices are in Dutch guilders

506. **Congrès français,** 1er–38e, de chirurgie. Procès-verbaux, Mémoires et discussions. 1886–1929. 38 vols. W. pl. and ill. 225.—
507. — Idem, 23e, 28e–30e, 32e, 33e, 35e. Paris 1910, 1919, 1920, Strasbourg 1921, Paris 1923, 1924, 1926. 7 vols. 15.—
508. — Idem, 41e. Paris 1932. Informations et rapports. 3.50
509. **Congreso español, 2°,** de cirugia. Madrid 1908. Actas. 8.50
510. **Congreso dental español, 3°.** Palma de Mallorca 1905. Actas. bound. 6.—
511. **Congres,** 4er–7er, der Deutschen dermatologischen Gesellschaft. 1894–1901. Verhandlungen. 4 vols. W. pl. 20.—
512. **Congreso ginecológico español.** Madrid 1888. Actas. bound. 7.50
513. **Congrès national** d'hygiène et de climatologie médicale de la Belgique et du Congo. Bruxelles 1897. Rapport avec le résumé des mémoires. Compte rendu des séances. 3 vols. 7.50
514. **Congrès** d'hygiène publique. Bruxelles 1851. Compte rendu des séances. Texte des résolutions votées. Pièces à l'appui. 2.50
515. **Congrès, 1er,** (de l') Alliance d'hygiène sociale. Arras 1904. [Travaux]. 4.—
Annales de l'alliance, etc. No. 1bis.
516. — 2e, (de l') Alliance d'hygiène sociale. Montpellier 1905. [Travaux]. 4.—
Annales de l'Alliance, etc. No. 3bis.
517. — 5e, (de l')Alliance d'hygiène sociale. Agen 1909. Plus spécialement sur l'hygiène rurale. Rapports et discussions. 4.—
518. — 7e, (de l') Alliance d'hygiène sociale. Roubaix 1911. Rapports et discussions. 4.—
519. **Congress,** 1er–32er, für innere Medicin. 1883–1921. Verhandlungen. 32 vols. W. tables of vols. I–XX. Tog. 33 vols. W. pl. 65.—
Added: **Verhandlungen** der ausserordentl. Tagung des Kongresses in Warschau. 1916.
520. — Idem, 49er. Wiesbaden 1937. Verhandlungen. bound. 25.—
521. **Congrès** de la lithiase urinaire. Vittel 1931. W. pl. 3.50
Revue médicale de l'Est. T. LIX, no. 21bis.
522. **Congrès français,** 13e, de médecine. Paris 1912. Rapports. 2.50
523. — 14e, de médecine. Bruxelles 1920. 11. Comptes rendus. Discussions et communications diverses. 2.—
524. — 20e, de médecine. Montpellier 1929. Comptes-rendus. Discussions et communications. Compte-rendu offic. et administratif. 2 vols. 4.—
Added: Idem. Rapport sur l'étiologie de la scarlatine par J. Cantacuzène.
525. **Congreso medico español.** Madrid 1864. Actas. bound. 6.—
526. — medico, 2°. Barcelona 1888. bound. (1060 pp.). 8.50
Congresos de ciencias médicas de Barcelona 1888. II.
527. **Congres, 1e–23e Nederlandsch natuur- en geneeskundig.** 1887–1931. Handelingen. 23 vols. W. pl. 75.—
528. — **3e Vlaamsch natuur- en geneeskundig.** Antwerpen 1899. Handelingen. 3.50
529. — **13e Vlaamsch natuur- en geneeskundig.** Brussel 1909. Handelingen. 3 parts. 3.50
530. — **14e Vlaamsch natuur- en geneeskundig.** Antwerpen 1910. Handelingen. Vol. III. 2.50
Le t. III est le plus important et est complet en soi-même. Les tom. I et II ne comprennent que les ff. prélimin. et les pp. 1 à 52.

Mart. Nijhoff, The Hague — Cat. No. 629

531. Congrès, 15e Vlaamsch natuur- en geneeskundig. Oostende 1911.
      Handelingen.   3.50
532. — 16e Vlaamsch natuur- en geneeskundig. Leuven 1912. Han-
      delingen. Vol. III.   2.50
533. — 17e Vlaamsch natuur- en geneeskundig. Gent 1913. Han-
      delingen.   3.50
534. Congrès belge, 2e, de neurologie et de psychiatrie. (Bruxelles 1906).
                                                                      3.—
535. Congres voor nijverheidshygiene en reddingswezen. Amsterdam
      1890. Verslag. 2 vols. bound.   3.—
536. Congreso español, 2°, de obstetricia, ginecologia y pediatria. Ma-
      drid 1911. Actas.   7.50
537. Congres, Nederlandsch, voor openbare gezondheidsregeling. Am-
      sterdam 1924. Praeadviezen en handelingen: Het wetsontwerp
      tegen besmettelijke ziekten.   1.25
538. Congres, Nederlandsch, voor openbare gezondheidsregeling. Am-
      sterdam 1937. Handelingen.   1.—
539. Kongress, 7er, der Deutschen Gesellschaft für orthopädische Chi-
      rurgie. Berlin 1908. Verhandlungen. W. 229 ill.   5.—
540. Congreso español, 3°, de oto-rino-laringologia. Sevilla 1910.
      Libro de actas.   6.—
541. Congresso pediatrico Italiano, 14°. Firenze 1931. Atti. In 2 vols.
                                                                      16.—
542. — pellagrologico italiano, 4°. Udine 1909. Atti.   4.—
543. Congrès national de pharmacie. Bruxelles 1895. Compte rendu.
      bound.   3.50
544. Congrès de phréniatrie et de neuropathologie. Anvers 1885.   4.—
545. Congrès de physiothérapie. Anvers 1920. Comptes rendus.   2.—
546. Congrès national scientifique. Prophylaxie des maladies pestilen-
      tielles exotiques. Anvers 1885. Comptes rendus et mémoires, etc.
                                                                      5.—
547. Congrès français, 1er, de stomatologie. Paris 1907. Comptes rendus.
                                                                      4.50
548. — 2e, de stomatologie. Paris 1911. Comptes rendus. bound.   4.50
549. — 7e, de stomatologie. Paris 1932. Compte rendu. Discours.
      Discussions des rapports. Communications.   6.—
550. — 8e, de stomatologie. Paris 1934. Compte rendu. Discours.
      Discussion des rapports. Communications.   4.50
551. Reunión, 1ra, de la Asociación española de urología. Madrid 1911.
      Temas ofic., comunicaciones y discusiones.   8.—
552. Congresso, 8°, della Società Italiana di urologia. Genova 1929.
      Atti. (9.—)   5.—
553. Congrès, 19e, 21e, 25e et 28e, (de l')Association française d'urologie.
      Paris 1919, Strasbourg 1921, Paris 1925, Paris 1928. Procès-ver-
      baux, Mémoires et Discussions. 4 vols. W. pl.   12.—
554. Tagung, 13e, der Gesellschaft für Verdauungs- und Stoffwechsel-
      krankheiten. 1937. Verhandlungen.   9.50

Prices are in Dutch guilders

LIVRES ANCIENS ET MODERNES

EN VENTE AUX PRIX MARQUÉS
CHEZ
MARTINUS NIJHOFF
La Haye, Lange Voorhout 9
adresse télégr.: Books Hague

Prices are in Dutch guilders. One guilder now about $ 0.55

RECENT ACQUISITIONS

Some divisions: **Anthropology — Australia — Balcan — Biographical dictionaries — Caricatures — China — Colonies — House of Orange — Jesuits — Marine — Netherlands — Railways**

1. **Wassenaer, Cl., en B. Lampe,** Historisch verhael al der ghedenckweerdichste geschiedenissen die hier en daer in Europa, als in Duijtsch-lant, Vranckrijck, Enghelant, Denemarcken, Spaengien, Hungarijen, Polen, Sweden, Moscovien, Sevenberghen, Wallachien, Moldavien, Turckijen en Neder-lant, van 1621–31 voorgevallen sijn. Amst. 1622–33. Vols. I–XX. bound in 7 vols. W. front. 4to. vellum. Gld. 1200.—

> Asher, nr. 330. This half yearly Register is of i m m e n s e i m p o r t- a n c e t o t h e h i s t o r y o f A m e r i c a; it contains above 150 „news of the day" relating to this part of the world, among which those on New Netherland are the more worthy of consideration, as they are the first printed reports on this country giving thousands of curious details and containing undoubtedly the most important and most curious of the first attempts at the colonisation of New-York. Further there will be found many news of the day relating to the Hollanders in Brasil and informations for colonists in Florida and Virginia, and also to historical events in all parts of the world.
> A complete set contains 21 vols., but the last vol. is of minor importance and has no interest for North America. Vols. I-IX are by far the most important for the history of that country.
> E x t r e m e l y s c a r c e.

---

2. **Alaska. — Burr, A.,** Alaska. Description of its rivers, volcanoes, big game hunters, mountain climbers; its pioneer settlements; its Indians; its romantic early history; the gold rush days, etc. Boston, 1919. W. map and 54 pl., of which 6 in coulours. cloth. 4.—
3. **Anabaptists. — Weill, A.,** Histoire de la guerre des Anabaptistes. Paris, 1874. 7.25
4. **— Westerbeek van Eerten B. Jzn., J. J.,** Anabaptisme en Calvinisme, 1531–1568. Kampen, 1905. 1.25

5. **Anthropology.** — **L'Anthropologie.** Paris, 1890–1932. T. 1–42. Av.
    table des tom. 1–20. 43 vol. Av. pl. et ill. dont 32 d. veau unif.,
    le reste en livr.   850.—
6. — **Anthropos.** Revue internat. d'ethnologie et de linguistique.
    Réd. P. W. Schmidt. Salzburg et St. Gabriel, 1906–37. Vol. 1–31,
    32, part 1–4. 27 vols. W. pl. 8 vols. hfcalf, 17 hfcloth, the remainder
    in parts.   800.—
    Complete set of this very valuable journal. All vols., except vol. 1, in the
    original imprint.
7. — **Beiträge** zur Anthropologie, Ethnographie und Archaeologie
    Niederl. Westindiens. Haarlem, 1904. Av. pl. 4to.   3.50
    Contient: **J. D. C. Schmeltz,** Ueber Sammlungen aus Niederl. West-
    indien und Surinam. — **C. Leemans,** Altertümer von Curaçao, Bonaire
    und Aruba. — **B. A. Koeze,** Schädel von Curaçao und Aruba.
    Mittheil. veröffentl. a. d. Niederl. Reichsmuseum für Völkerkunde.
    Série II, no. 9.
8. — **Bolzano, B.,** Ueber das Verhältnis der beiden Volksstämme in
    Böhmen. Wien, 1894.   3.—
    Première edition.
9. — **Bulletin et mémoires de la Société d'anthropologie de Bruxelles.**
    Brux. 1883–1936. T. 1–51, dont 32 tom. en 18 vol. d. rel., le reste br.
                                                                                         250.—
10. — **Bulletins de la Société d'anthropologie de Paris** (*dès l'année* 1900:)
    Bulletins et Mémoires. Paris, 1860–1930. 1re–7e séries. 70 tom.
    Av. pl. et figg. dont 30 vol. rel., le reste br. et en livr.   575.—
    En grande partie epuisé et très rare.
    Un titre et 2 tables manquent.
11. — **Burdach, K. F.,** Anthropologie. Stuttgart, 1837. cart.   6.—
12. — **Cabanès, P. J. G.,** Ueber die Verbindung des Physischen und
    Moralischen in dem Menschen. A. d. Franz. m. Abhandl. üb. die
    Grenzen der Physiologie und der Anthropologie von L. H. Jakob.
    Halle, 1804. 2 vol. d. veau.   20.—
    Traduction rare.
13. — **Congrès internat.,** 2e, 4e–12e, d'anthropologie et d'archéologie
    préhistoriques. Compte rendu. Paris, Copenhague, etc. 1867–1900.
    12 tom. 11 vol. Av. pl. toile.   100.—
    2e, Paris 1867; 4e, Copenhague 1869; 5e, Bologne 1871; 6e, Bruxelles
    1872; 7e, Stockholm 1874. 2 vols.; 8e, Budapest 1876; 9e, Lisbonne 1880;
    10e, Paris 1889; 11e Moscou, 1892. 2 tom. 1 vol.; 12e, Paris 1900.
    Série très rare. Du ser Congrès ne pas un compte rendu a paru.
14. — — Idem, 5e. Bologne 1871. Av. pl. *Très rare.*   18.—
15. — — Idem, 6e. Bruxelles 1872. Av. 90 cartes et pl. rel.   7.50
16. — — Idem, 7e. Stockholm 1874. 2 vol. Av. cartes et ill.   10.—
17. — — Idem, 8e. Budapest 1876. 2 tom. 3 vol. Av. cartes, pl. et
    ill. d. veau.   15.—
18. — — Idem, 9e. Lisbonne 1880. Av. pl. d. veau.   10.—
19. — — Idem, 11e. Moscou 1892. 2 tom. 1 vol. Av. ill. rel.   12.—
20. — — Idem, 12e. Paris 1900. Av. pl.   8.50
21. — — Idem, 15e. Portugal 1930, Paris 1931. 2 vol. Av. pl.   10.—
    4e et 5e Session de l'Institut Internat. d'anthropologie.
22. — — Idem, 16e. Bruxelles 1935. Av. ill.   12.—
    6e Session de l'Institut Internat. d'anthropologie.
23. — **Congrès internat.,** 3e, d'anthropologie criminelle. Bruxelles 1892.
    Actes. Biologie et sociologie. Brux. 1893.   6.—

24. **Anthropology.** — **Congrès internat.**, 4e, d'anthropologie criminelle. Genève 1897. Comptes rendus des travaux. Genève, 1897. toile. 6.—
25. — — Idem, 5e. Amsterdam 1901. Compte rendu des traveaux. Amst. 1901. Av. ill. d. chagr. 14.—
26. — — Idem, 6e. Turin 1906. Comptes rendus. Milan 1908. Av. pl. 15.—
27. — **Congrès internat.** des sciences anthropologiques. Paris 1878. Comptes rendus sténograph. Paris, 1880. 7.50.
28. — **Congrès internat.**, Ier, des sciences anthropologiques et ethnologiques. Londres 1934. Compte rendu. London, 1934. 15.—
29. — — Idem, 2e. Copenhague 1938. Compte rendu. Copenhague, 1939. 17.50
30. — **Diefenbach, L.**, Origines Europae. Die alten Völker Europas mit ihren Sippen und Nachbarn. Frankfurt, 1861. d. rel. 3.—
31. — **Dixon, R. B.**, The racial history of man. N. York, 1923. W. 44 pl. cloth. 4.50
   I. Europe. (British isles and Scandinavia; the Jews and gipsies, etc.). — II. Africa. — III. Asia. — IV. Oceania. — V. North America. — VI South America. — etc.
32. — **Ethnographie et anthropologie.** — [Collection d'écrits en allemand, anglais et français]. 1876–1908. Ens. 120 pièces. Av. pl. et ill. 4to et 8vo. *Pour la plupart des tirages à part et des nos de périodiques.* 45.—
   Contient e.a.: **M. Bartels**, Schädel-Masken aus Neu-Britannien, besond. mit Kopfverletzung. — **J. Bellucci**, Catalogue descriptif d'une collection d'amulettes italiennes à l'expos. de Paris, 1889. — **H. M. Bernelot Moens**, Wahrheit. Uber die Abstammung des Menschen. — **D. I. Bushnell**, Virginia from early records. — **K. Ertl**, Heimatskunde von Oberklee. — **F. Heger**, Verschwundene Altmexikan. Kostbarkeiten des XVI Jahrhunderts. — **F. S. Krauss**, Vidirlijic Ahmo's Brautfahrt. — **L. Leiner**, Vom Pfahlbautenwesen am Bodensee. — **A. Maass**, Die primitive Kunst der Mentawei-Insulaner. — **Z. Nuttall**, A penitential rite of the ancient Mexicans. — **K. Weule**, Die Eidechse als Ornament in Afrika. — **N. Puccioni**, Delle deformazioni e mutilazioni artificiali etniche più in uso. — **S. H. Ray**, Compar. vocabulary of the dialects of British New Guinea. — etc.
33. — **Fritsch, G.**, Die Eingeborenen Süd-Afrika's ethnograph. und anatomisch. Breslau, 1872. Av. 20 pl. et ill. gr. in-8vo. Av. atlas de 30 pl. 4to. Ens. 2 vol. toile orig. (1 pl. de l'atlas est montée). 25.— Important ouvrage, estimé et épuisé.
34. — **Hagen, B.**, Kopf- und Gesichtstypen. Ostasiatischer und Melanesischer Völker. Stuttgart, 1906. 50 planches se dépliant av. texte. fol.-obl. d. rel. (60.—) 20.— II. Abschnitt: Vorder-Indier.
35. — **Heinroth, J. Chr. A.**, Lehrbuch der Anthropologie. Lpz. 1822. cart. 5.—
36. — **Kant, I.**, Anthropologie in pragmatischer Hinsicht. 2e Aufl. Königsberg, 1800. cart. 1.75
37. — **Krause, K. C. F.**, Vorlesungen über die psychische Anthropologie. Göttingen, 1848. 6.—
38. — **Laing, S.**, Human origins. London, 1892. Av. ill. toile. 2.50
39. — **Le Cat**, Traité de la couleur de la peau humaine en général, de celle des nègres en particulier, et de la métamorphose d'une de

ces couleurs en l'autre, soit de naissance, soit accidentellement.
Amst. 1765. Av. front. d'après Gravelot. veau. 12.—

40. **Anthropology.** — **Lundborg, H.,** Die Rassenmischung beim Menschen. 's-Grav. 1931. Av. 5 pl. (14.—) 8.—
Tirage à part de 221 pp. de „Bibliographia genetica".

41. — **d'Omalius d'Halloy, J. J.,** Des races humaines ou éléments d'ethnographie. 5e éd. Brux. 1869. Av. 1 pl. lith. color. 2.—

42. — **Pruys van der Hoeven, C.,** Anthropologisch onderzoek. 2e dr. Leiden, 1854. 4 vol. toile. 2.—
Contient e.a. de courtes biographies de médecins et de philosophes (Baco, Harvey, Sydenham, Galenus, Hippocrates etc.).

43. — **Rachel, H.,** Geschichte der Völker und Kulturen, vom Urbeginn bis heute. Berlin, 1920. cart. 4.—

44. — **Review, The anthropological.** London, 1863–67. Vol. I-V. 5 vol. boards. 10.—

45. — **Revue d'anthropologie.** Publ. sous la dir. de P. Broca, P. Topinard e.a. Paris, 1872–89. Série I, 6 vol; série II, 8 vol.; série III, 4 vol. Ens. 18 vol. d. veau unif. 300.—
Tout ce qui a paru.

46. — **Revue mensuelle de l'Ecole d'anthropologie de Paris** (*plus tard*: Revue anthropologique). Fondé par A. Hovelacque. Paris, 1891–1929. Année 1–39. Av. tables des années 1891–1910. 41 vol. Av. pl. et figg. dont 29 vol. d. rel., le reste en livr. 800.—

47. — **Rodier, G.,** Antiquité des races humaines. Paris, 1864. d. veau.
1.75
Chronologie des Egyptiens, des Grecs, des Hébreux, des Indous, etc. Histoire. Egypte, de l'an 18790 à l'an 332 av. J. C. etc., etc. Textes justific.

48. — **Semple, E. Ch.,** Influences of geographic environment. On the basis of Ratzel's system of anthropo-geography. N. York, 1911. W. maps and pl. cloth. 2.50

49. — **Steffens, H.,** Anthropologie. Breslau, 1822. 2 vols. 6.—

50. — **Stuart, M.,** De mensch, zooals hij voorkomt op den bekenden aardbol. Z. Boemel, 1818. 6 vol. Av. front. color. et 43 pl., dont 41 color., par L. Partman d'après J. Kuyper. cart. orig. 15.—
Le t. III légèr. atteint d'humidité.

51. — **Techet, C.,** Völker, Vaterländer und Fürsten. Beitr. z. Entwicklung Europas. München, 1913. Av. pl. et ill. 3.50
Langschädel und Kurzschädel. — Die Slaven. — Rassenmischung und das Europäertum. — Ruszland, die Magyaren und die Osmanen. — etc.

52. — **Vierkandt, A.,** Naturvölker und Kulturvölker. Lpz. 1896. *Très rare.* 15.—

53. — **Waitz, Th.,** Anthropologie der Naturvölker. Lpz. 1859–72. 6 vol. d.veau. 75.—
Tous les volumes en impression originale.

54. **Australia.** — (**Brosses, Ch. de,**) Histoire des navigations aux terres australes. Paris, 1756. 2 vol. Av. 7 cartes se dépliant et 1 carte ajoutée. 4to. veau marbré, dos dor. *Bel ex.* 60.—

55. — (**Claret de Fleurieu, Ch. P.**), Découvertes des François, en 1768 et 1769, dans le sud-est de la Nouvelle Guinée, préc. de l'abrégé histor. des navigations des Espagnols dans les mêmes parages. Paris, 1790. Av. 12 cartes et pl. repliées. 4to. veau. (Rel. frottée). 20.—

Prices are in guilders

56. **Australia. — Cust, R.,** Les races et les langues de l'Océanie. Trad.
p. A. L. Pinart. Paris, 1888. pet. in-8vo. veau. 2.—

57. **— Journal des Museum Godeffroy.** Geograph., ethnograph. und
naturwissenschaftl. Mittheilungen. Hrsg. von R. Bergh, L. Friede-
richsen, J. Kubary, G. Semper, u. A. Hamburg, 1873–1910. 6 vols.
W. 4 maps, 98 pl., 17 of which coloured, and 180 fine coloured pl.
of Australian fishes. 450.—
This highly valuable publication is devoted to the ethnography, zoology
and geography of Australia and the Pacific.
All published. Out of print and becoming scarce.

58. **— Malinowski, B.,** The family among the Australian aborigenes.
Sociolog. study. London, 1913. toile. 7.50

59. **— Nicholas, J. L.,** Narrative of a voyage to New Zealand in the
years 1814 and 1815. London, 1817. 2 vol. Av. 2 front., 2 cartes et
2 pl. cart. orig., n. r. *Très bel ex.* 30.—
Edition originale.

60. **— Royal Society of Van Diemensland** (*later*: of Tasmania). Papers
and proceedings. Hobart Town, 1848–59. Vol. 1–III, 1–2. (Complete). — (*Continued by*:) **Monthly notices** of papers and proceedings of the Royal Society of Tasmania (*later:* Papers and proceedings). Hobart Town, 1863, 1865, 1872–1902. — Tog. 33 vols. W.
pl. 450.—
Contains primarily contributions on zoology, botany and geology, but
also important articles on Tasmania's history and ethnography. Very
scarce. Between 1860—1862 nothing was published.

61. **— Tasman, A. Jz.,** Journal of his discovery of Van Diemens Land
and New Zealand, in 1642. W. documents rel. to his exploration
of Australia in 1644, being facsimiles of the original ms. W. Engl.
transl. ed. by J. E. Heeres, and observat., made with the com-
pass on the voyage by W. van Bemmelen. Amst. 1898. Av. cartes,
pl. et figg. fol. vél., tr. dor. *Epuisé.* 135.—
Facsimilé du ms. original, orné de nombr. cartes et dessins par Tasman lui-même, sur 195 pp., donnant une exacte reproduction photo-
lithogr. du célèbre journal. Accomp. d'une traduction anglaise sur 59 pp.
et de 162 pp., occupées par une histoire de la vie et des travaux de T.
par Heeres. C'est la première relation exacte de tout ce qui concerne ce
célèbre navigateur.

62. **— Twain, Mark,** Letters from the Sandwich Islands. Introd. by
G. E. Dane. Stanford University, 1938. W. ill. cloth. 6.—

63. **-- Waitz, Th.,** Anthropologie der Naturvölker. V, 2. Die Mikro-
nesier, und Nortwestl. Polynesier. Fortges. von G. Gerland. Lpz.
1870. 1.50

64. **— Wilson, C. A.,** The Empire's junior partner (New-Zealand).
London, 1926. Av. ill. toile. **— The peopling of Australia** by W. E.
Agar, H. Benham a.o. Melbourne, 1928. d. rel. — **New Zealand
Affairs** by A. T. Ngata, G. H. Scholefield, W. Nash a.o. Christchurch,
1929. d. rel. — Ens. 3 vol. 3.50

65. **Balcan. — Grimm, A. Th. von,** Wanderungen nach Südosten.
Berlin, 1855–56. 3 vol. cart. 1.75
I. Die Taurische Halbinsel. — II. Die Oriental. Frage, geschichtl. ent-
wickelt. Der Bosporus und die fränkischen Vorstädte. — III. Constanti-
nopel.

66. **— Hobhouse, J. C.,** Journey through Albania a.o. provinces of

Mart. Nijhoff, The Hague — Cat. No. 630

Turkey in Europe and Asia, to Constantinople, 1809 and 1810.
London, 1813. W. front., maps and 17 coloured pl. 4to. boards. 25.—

67. **Balcan.** — **Iorga, N.**, Roemeensche kunst en letterkunde. Synthet.
vergelijkingen. Vert. van J. Gaster en P. Valkhof. Maastricht,·
1932. Av. 69 pl.   3.—

68. — **Leven, Het ellendigh,** der Turcken, Moscoviters en Chinesen,
aende christenheyt vertoont. Ofte korte beschryvinge van yder in
't bysonder zijn regeringh, handel en wandel, etc. en wat wreet-
heydt zy ontrent haer selfs e. a. natien gebruycken. 's-Grav., J.
Tongerloo, 1663. Av. grav. sur le titre, répétée dans le texte, 1 pl.
hors et une dans le texte. 4to. d. vél.   20.—

69. — **Meneses, L. de,** Exemplar de virtudes morales de Jorge Castrio-
to, llamado Scanderbeg, principe de los Epirotas, y Albaneses.
Lisboa, 1688. 4to. calf.   15.—

70. — **Paton, A. A.**, Highlands and islands of the Adriatic, incl.
Dalmatia, Croatia, the southern provinces of the Austrian empire.
London, 1849. 2 vols. W. map and pl. cloth.   6.—

71. — **((Sommerlatt, C. V.)**, Beschreibung der Kaiserstadt Constan-
tinopel, ihrer Umgebungen, Sitten und Gebräuche. Nebst Anhang,
die türkische Festungsstadt Schumla darstellend. Coblentz, 1829.
W. maps, plan and pl.   3.50

72. — **Strangford, Viscountess,** The eastern shores of the Adriatic in
1863. With a visit to Montenegro. London, 1864. W. front. and
4 coloured pl. cloth. (Back damaged).   4.50
        Southern Albania, A few words on Corfu politics, Ragusa, Montenegro,
        on Northern Albania, Dalmatia, etc.

73. — **Welcker, F. G.**, Tagebuch einer Griechischen Reise (1842).
Berlin, 1865. 2 vol.   1.75

74. — **Wencel, K.**, Der Kampf der Südslawen um Freiheit und Einheit.
Frankfurt, 1925. cloth. (9.—)   2.50

75. — **Westrik, J.**, Konstantinopel, Smyrna, Suez-kanaal, Jerusalem.
Amst. 1870. Av. portr. de F. de Lesseps et 6 pl. color. cart. 1.50

76. — **Wiebel, K. W. M.**, Die Insel Kephalonia und die Meermühlen
von Argostoli. Hamburg, 1873. Av. carte. 4to. cart.   1.50

77. **Baltische Monatschrift.** Riga, 1859–1915. Year 1–56, 57, nrs. 1–6.
Tog. 78 vols. in 80. of which 52 vols. bound.   500.—
        The principal baltic journal, contain. articles on the history, the lite-
        rature, the folklore, law, economic and social sciences, etc. especially
        relat. to the Baltics (and Russia).
        Very rare in complete state. Pp. 185–188 of vol. 48 are lacking to all
        copies, being suppressed by the censor.
        The years 1914–1915 were publ. under the title: ,,Deutsche Monatschrift''.
        After 1915 this periodical was discontinued, but a new series started 1928.

78. **Bauer, Br.**, Vollständ. Geschichte der Partheikämpfe in Deutschland während der Jahre 1842–1846. Charlottenburg, 1847. 2 vol.
d. rel.   12.—

79. **Biographical dictionaries.** — **Aa, A. J. van der,** Biographisch woordenboek der Nederlanden, bevatt. levensbeschrijvingen van personen, die zich in ons vaderland hebben vermaard gemaakt, voort-
gezet d. K. J. R. van Harderwijk en G. D. J. Schotel. M. Suppl.
Haarlem, 1851–79. 21 vols. in 27. Hfcalf.   250.—
        The best Dutch biographical dictionary.

                        Prices are in guilders

80. **Biographical dictionaries. — Aa, A. J. van der,** Nieuw biografiesch, anthologiesch en kritiesch woordenboek van Nederlandsche dichters. Onder medew. van Bodel Nyenhuis, Da Costa, Schotel, enz. Amst. 1864. 3 vol. Av. portrait. cart. 15.—

81. — **Acta Sanctorum Belgii** selecta, tum ex monumentis necdum in Bollandiano opere editis, tum ex illo opere coll. J. Ghesquierus. Brux. 1783–94. 6 vols. W. portr. and pl. 4to. calf. 65.—
Scarce with the 6th volume.

82. — **Ader, J.,** Plutarque des Pays-Bas, ou vies des hommes illustres de ce royaume, av. introd. histor. Brux. 1828. 3 vol. Av. portr. cart. 7.50

83. — **Andreae, V.,** Bibliotheca belgica: de Belgis vita scriptisque clariss. praem. topograph. Belgiae totius s. Germ. Infer. descriptio. Ed. renov. et 4a parte auct. Lovan., J. Zegers, 1643. 4to. calf. 30.—

84. — **Baier, J. J.,** Biographiae professorum medicinea qui in academia Altorfina unquam vixerunt. Norimb. 1728. Av. 15 portr. (200 pp.). *Très rare.*

— **Linden, J. A. van der,** Lindenius renovatur, sive ... de scriptis medicis. Contin. a G. A. Mercklino. Norimb. 1686. Av. front. (1156 + 162 pp.).
Grande bibliographie médicale.
En 1 vol. 4to. d. vél. 60.—

85. — **Becdelièvre, De,** Biographie Liégoise ou précis histor. et chronolog. de toutes les personnes qui se sont rendues célèbres dans l'ancien pays de Liège, les duchés de Limbourg et de Bouillon, la ville de Maestricht, etc. Bibliographie Liégoise. Liège, 1836, 37. 2 vol. d. veau. 15.—

86. — **Biographie** des hommes célèbres, des savans, des artistes et des littérateurs du Dépt. de la Somme. Amiens, 1835, 38. 2 tom. Av. suppl. En 2 vol. Av. portraits. 6.—

87. — **Biographie générale, Nouvelle,** depuis les temps les plus reculés jusqu'à nos jours. Publ. par Firmin Didot sous la direction de Hoefer. Paris, 1854–66. 46 tom. 23 vol. veau. 90.—

88. — **Biographie nationale.** Publ. par l'Académie Royale des sciences, des lettres et des beaux-arts de Belgique. Brux. 1866–1938. 27 tom. 13 vol. toile et 1 br. 150.—
Cet important ouvrage est maintenant terminé. Un volume conprenant une table générale est sous presse.

89. — **Biographie universelle,** ancienne et moderne (Michaud). Paris, 1811–28. 52 vol. d. veau unif. 40.—

90. — — Même ouvrage Av. le Suppl. (A-Vil). Paris, Michaud, 1811–62. 85 vol. d. veau. (Dos endomm.). 80.—
Tout ce qui a paru.

91. — — Même ouvrage. Nouv. éd. publ. par Michaud. Paris, 1854–65. 45 vol. d. veau. 90.—

92. — **Biographie, Allgemeine Deutsche.** Lpz. 1875–1912. 55 vols. W. index. Tog. 56 vols. Hfcalf. *Fine copy.* 225.—

93. — **Burman, C.,** Traiectum eruditum virorum doctrina inlustrum, qui in urbe Traiecto et regione Trajectensi nati sunt, s. ibi habitarunt, vitas, fata et scripta exhibens. Ultr., J. A. Paddenburg, 1738. 4to. vél. 10.—

94. **Biographical dictionaries.** — **Feller, F. X. de,** Biographie univ. ou dictionnaire histor. des hommes qui se sont fait un nom. Nouv. éd., revue et continuée jusqu'en 1838. Paris, 1838–39. 5 vol. d. veau. 15.—

94a. — **Foppens, J. F.,** Bibliotheca belgica s. virorum in Belgio vita scriptisque illustrium catalogus, librorumque nomenclatura cont. scriptt. à Val. Andrea, A. Miraeo, F. Sweertio, al., recens. usque ad ann. 1680. Brux. 1739. 2 vols. W. 144 portr. 4to. calf. 65.—

95. — **Galerie historique** des contemporains, ou nouvelle biographie . . des hommes morts ou vivans, de toutes les nations, fin du 18e siècle et au commencement de celui-ci, leurs écrits, leurs actions, etc. Av. 2 Suppl. Brux. 1818–26. 10 vol., dont 8 veau marbré, dos dor. (Les dos de 3 vol. légèr. endomm.). 25.—
Par P. L. P. Jullian pour la partie politique, Ph. Lesbroussart pour la partie littéraire et G. van Lennep pour ce qui concerne la Hollande.
Ex. complet avec les 2 Suppléments.

96. — **Glasius, B.,** Godgeleerd Nederland. Biographisch woordenboek van Nederl. godgeleerden. 's-Hert. 1851–56. 3 vol. 12.—

97. — **Immerzeel Jr., J.,** De levens en werken der Hollandsche en Vlaamsche kunstschilders, beeldhouwers, graveurs en bouwmeesters van het begin der 15e eeuw tot heden. Uitgeg. d. C. H. en C. Immerzeel. Amst. 1842–43. 3 vols. in 1. W. portr. and monograms. Hfbound. 40.—

98. — **Joecher, Chr. G.,** Compendiöses Gelehrten Lexikon. 3. Aufl. Lpz. 1733. 2 vol. veau. 10.—

99. — **Kobus, J. C.,** en **W. de Rivecourt,** Biographisch woordenboek van Nederland. Nieuwe uitg. Arnhem, 1886. 3 vol. toile. 5.—

100. — **Levensbeschrijving** van eenige voorname meest Nederl. mannen en vrouwen. Amst., P. Conradi, 1777–83. 10 tom. 9 vol. d. veau. 18.—

101. — **Levensbeschrijving, Korte,** der Nederl. vorsten, helden en vermaarde mannen, geschikt naar de eeuwen waarin ze geleefd hebben. Amst. 1766. 2 vol. veau, dos ornés. 12.—

102. — **Loosjes, J.,** Naamlijst van predikanten, hoogleeraren en proponenten der Luthersche kerk in Nederland. Biographie en bibliographie. 's-Grav. 1925. toile. 3.50

103. — **Mancheño y Olivares, M.,** Galería de Arcobricenses ilustres. Arcos de la Frontera, 1892. 5.—
Biographies of about 75 persons born at Arcos de la Frontera.

104. — **Mathieu, A.,** Biographie montoise. Mons, 1848. d. veau. 5.—

105. — **Nagler, G. K.,** Neues allgemeines Künstler-Lexikon oder Nachrichten von dem Leben und den Werken der Maler, Bildhauer, Baumeister, Kupferstecher.... Medailleure, etc. 2e Aufl. Unveränd. Abdr. der ersten Aufl. 1835–52. Linz, 1904–14. 25 vols. Hfbound. 75.—
This reimpression, (printed on better paper than the original edition) is not to be confounded with the inferior anastatical reprint of 1925.

106. — **(Nicéron, J. P., P. F. Oudin, J. B. Michaudt** et **C. P. Goujet,** Mémoires pour servir à l'histoire des hommes illustres dans la république des lettres. Av. un catalogue raisonné de leurs ouvrages.

Prices are in guilders

Paris, 1726–45. 43 tom. 44 vol. 12mo. veau fauve, dos dor. (*Simier-Duroi*). *Bel ex.* 200.—
Cet ouvrage très recherché renferme un grand nombre de notices curieuses, des renseignements précieux puisés à des sources trop peu explorées. La partie bibliograph. surtout mérite d'être fréquemment consultée. Les exx. complets de 43 vol. sont extrêmement rares.
Exemplaire fort précieux en ce qu'il a appartenu au très savant abbé Papillon, auteur de la ,,Bibliothèque des auteurs de Bourgogne'' (dont il porte la signature) et qu'il est chargé de notes manuscr. de sa main, la plupart instructives et intéressantes.

107. **Biographical dictionaries. — Paz–Soldan, J. P.**, Diccionario biografico de Peruanos contemporaneos. Lima, 1917. 7.50

108. **— Plutarchus,** 't Leven der doorluchtige Griecken ende Romeynen. Wt de Griecsche sprake d. J. Amyot. Verduyscht d. A. v(an) Zuÿlen) v(an) N(euivelt). Delft, A. G. van Beyeren, 1644. Av. front. fol. d. veau. (Rel. endomm.). 25.—
Deuxième édition de la première traduction néerland. complète des Vies de Plutarque. La première parut en 1603.

109. **— (Rossi, J. Victor)**, Pinacotheca imaginum illustrium doctrinae vel ingenii laude virorum qui, auctore superstite, diem suum obierunt (a. J. Nicio). Colon. Agripp. 1645. 2 parties en 1 vol. Av. titre gravé et portrait. pet. in-8vo. vél. 28.—
On y trouve des biographies de plusieurs personnes que l'on cherchera vainement ailleurs.

110. **— Samazeuilh, J. F.**, Biographie de l'arrondissement de Nérac. Nérac, 1857. pet. in-8vo. d. rel. 3.50
Le titre est remplacé par la couverture.

111. **— Seyn, E. de,** Dictionnaire biographique des sciences, des lettres et des arts en Belgique. Brux. 1935, 36. 2 vol. Av. de nombr. pl. et portr. dans le texte. gr. in-4to. d. veau. 36.—

112. **— Thieme, W.,** und **F. Becker,** Allgemeines Lexikon der bildenden Künstler von der Antike bis zur Gegenwart. Unter Mitwirk. von 300 Fachgelehrten. Lpz. 1907–38. Vol. 1–32 (A-Theodotos). 32 vols. orig. hfcalf. (1385.—) 700.—

113. **— Vasari, G.,** Le vite de piu eccellenti architetti, pittori et scultori Italiani. Firenze, 1550. 3 parties. 2 vol. 4to. veau. 150.—
Première édition de cet ouvrage célèbre, contenant des détails qui sont omis dans les éditions suivantes.
Nom sur le titre, pour le reste un bel ex. bien conservé.

114. **— Waller, F. G.,** Biographisch woordenboek van Noord Nederlandsche graveurs. Bewerkt d. W. R. Juynboll. 's-Grav. 1938. W. 61 beautiful portraits. cloth. 26.—
This work forms an indispensable supplement especially to Thieme-Becker's Künstlerlexicon. It does not contain a list of the works of the artists, but gives exact details concerning all that is to be found in archives a.o. sources; it fixes f.i. exact dates and mentions the technics used by the artists. As to the modern engravers, several of which are among the living still, the here given material is almost wholly new.

115. **— Weyerman, J. C.,** Levens-beschrijvingen der Nederl. kunstschilders en -schilderessen. 's-Grav. 1729. 3 vol. Av. front. et 102 portr. 4to. d. veau. 20.—
Sans le t. IV.

116. **— Wie is dat?** Naamlijst van ongeveer 4000 bekende personen op elk gebied in het Kon. der Nederlanden. Met biograf. aanteeken.,

opgave hunner voornaamste werken, adressen, enz., enz. 4e uitg.
's-Grav. 1938. toile. 6.50
Le ,,Who's who" des Pays-Bas.

117. **Biographical dictionaries. — Witsen Geysbeek, P. G.**, Biograph.,
antholog. en critisch woordenboek der nederd. dichters. Amst.
1821–27. 6 vol. 15.—

118. **— Wolff, O. L. B.**, Encyclopädie der deutschen Nationalliteratur.
Biograph.-krit. Lexicon der Dichter und Prosaisten, nebst Proben
aus ihren Werken. Lpz. 1835–47. 8 tom. 5 vol. pet. in-fol. d. veau. 7.50

119. **— Woordenboek, Biographisch**, van Protestantsche godgeleerden
in Nederland. Onder red. van J. P. de Bie, J. Loosjes, J. Lindeboom
e.a. 's-Grav. 1903–39. T. I–IV, V, 1–7 (A-Lansbergen). 4 vol.
toile (V, 1–5 br.). (98.30) 56.80
Cet ouvrage contient les biographies des théologiens protestants néerland.
dès la Réforme jusqu'à nos jours. Chaque biographie est suivi d'une liste des
ouvragesde la personne décrite et d'une indication de la littérature sur elle.

120. **— Woordenboek, Nieuw Nederlandsch biographisch.** Onder red. van
P. C. Molhuysen, P. J. Blok en F. K. H. Kossmann. Leiden, 1911-
38. 10 vols. Hfcalf. (150.—) 90.—
National biographical dictionary of the Netherlands.

121. **— Wurzbach, A. von**, Niederländisches Künstler-Lexikon. Wien,
1907–11. 3 vols. in 5. Hfcalf. 75.—
The original imprint. Very fine copy.

122. **— Wurzbach, C. von**, Biographisches Lexikon des Kaiserthums
Oesterreich enthaltend die Lebensskizzen der denkwürdigen Personen, welche seit 1750 in den österreich. Kronländern geboren
wurden oder darin gelebt und gewirkt haben. Wien, 1856–91.
60 vols. Hfcloth. 425.—
All vols. in the original imprint.

123. **Bolshevism. — Champney, E. W.**, and **F.**, Romance of Russia. From
rurik to bolshevik. N. York, 1922. W. 47 pl. cloth. (12.60) 4.—

124. **— Russische Korrespondenz.** No pl. 1920–22. 3 years. 6 vols. in 5.
With 1 vol ,,Beilage" 1921–22. Tog. 6 vols. W. maps and numer.
coloured and plain pl. roy. 8vo. Hfcloth. 250.—
All published. The leading journal of bolshevism and of the greatest
rarity. Nr. 1–4 of vol. I (= pp. 1–100) are missing.

125. **Brailsford, H. N.**, Hoe lang nog? Een boek over deze verdwaasde
wereld en haar behoefte aan eenheid. U. h. Eng. d. W. van Rave-
steyn. Zutphen, 1929. (4.50) 1.50
Versailles. — Genève. — Locarno. — Pan-Europa. — Moskou en de
eenheid van Azië. — Pan-Amerika. — Ontwapening. — etc.

126. **Caricatures, Satyre. — Antonio Maria.** Lisboa, 1879–84. 6 vol.
Av. de nombr. caricatures (qq. années av. pl. color.). gr. in-4to.
cart. orig. ill. 60.—
Collection dès le commencement de cette revue satyrique spirituelle,
illustrée par les meilleurs caricaturistes portugais du temps.
Pour la continuation voir le no. 133a.

127. **— L'Aassiette au beurre.** Paris, 1901–18 mars 1911. Nos. 1–520. En
10 vol. gr. in 4to. d. veau.
Journal satyrique avec des ill. par Steinlen, Veber, Jossot, Villon,
Hénaulty le Petit. Vogel, Jeannot, Willette, Léandre, Roubille, Mikhael,
Leal de Carama, Herman Paul, Caran d'Arche, 1bels e.a. Il fut continué
jusqu'à 1912, mais il avait alors perdu beaucoup de sa valeur artistique.
Collection rare.

Prices are in guilders

128. **Caricatures, Satyre. — Chat noir.** Organe des intérêts de Mont-
martre. Dir. Rodolph Salis, réd. Emile Goudeau, Alphonse Allais
e.a. Paris, 1882–89. Année 1–8 (= nos. 1-415). Av. une foule d'ill.
par Willette, Gill, Caran d'Ache, Steinlen, Bombled e.a. fol. Rel.
en 4 vol. d. rel. 45.—
    Célèbre journal montmartrois.

129. — — **[Ombres chinoises]** données au Chat Noir ou publ. à la même
époque (vers 1890). Musique de Fragerolle, Vieu, Mulder, Alexandre
Georges, dessins de Rivière, Fraipont, Uzès, Métivet, Bombled,
etc. Paris, (v. 1890). 16 vols. 4to-obl. orig. boards, 3 sewed,
preserved covers. 60.—
    We believe this collection is complete. It contains: La tentation de Saint
    Antoine. Féerie p. H. Rivière. Musique p. A. Tinchant et G. Fragerolle. —
    Aladin. Ombres chinoises p. L. Métivet. Musique p. J. Vieu. — La belle
    au bois dormant. Féerie chantée p. L. Métivet. Musique p. J. Vieu. —
    Lourdes. Légende mystique p. G. Fragerolle et Desveaux-Vérité. Musique
    p. G. Fragerolle. — Le roi de Thulé. Légende du Nord p. Desveaux-Vérité.
    Musique p. J. Fragerolle. — La marche à l'Etoile. 2 albums, les 2 versions
    différentes. — Les Boers p. L. Bombled. Musique p. J. Mulder, etc.
    In the eighties and nineties the ,,Chat Noir" at Paris was a famous
    ,,Cabaret" where Aristide Bruant and others took the lead. Besides their
    ,,chansons" they also brought into fashion the ,,Ombres chinoises" cleverly
    cut in cartoon, and projected on linen. They were very much ,,en vogue"
    for a certain time and the books reproducing some of them must have
    been quite popular. It is a very scarce collection that we offer here, it
    is a charming representation of a kind of entertainment in that period.

130. — **Cri de Paris, Le.** Paris, 31 janv. 1897–19 janv. 1919. 22 années.
Av. de nombr. ill. 4to. dont les 16 premières années rel. en d. bas.
rouge, les autres en fasc. 120.—
    Hebdomadaire illustrée. En ses 1.138 fascicules, c'est toute la ,,Petite
    Histoire" de Paris racontée, tant au point de vue politique que mondain
    et théatral. La couverture de chaque no. est illustrée d'un dessin par Nau-
    din, Truchet, Ricardo Florès, Jehan Testevuide, e.a.
    Tout ce qui a paru. 4 nos. manquent (842, 850, 863 et 1.089).

131. — **Don Quichotte, Le.** Journal satyrique illustré. Paris, 1874–87.
Année 1-14. En 7 vol. Av. de nombr. pl. caricatur. en couleurs.
fol. d. veau. 35.—
    Les titres et les tables des t. 1–10 manquent (parus?).

131a. — **Parodia, A.** Lisboa, 1900–07. 8 years in 7 vols. W. numerous
caricatural ill. in colours and plain. roy. 4to. orig. ill. cloth. 70.—
    Complete collection of this satyrical weekly.

132. — **Parodie, La.** Publ. p. A. Gill. Paris, 4 juin 1869–16 janv. 1870.
Année I, II, nos. 1–21. Av. de nombr. ill., en partie en couleurs. En
1 vol. fol. d. rel., couv. conservée. 12.50

132a. — **Patriota, Supplemento burlesco do.** Lisboa, 1847–53. 540 differ.
nrs. W. satyrical lith. pl. and ill. In 1 vol. fol. hfcalf. (Back
damaged). 25.—

133. — **Pinto, M.,** Don Pirlone à Roma. Memorie di un Italiano dal
1° Sett. 1848. al 21 Dec. 1850. Torino, 1850. 3 vol. Av. 306 pl. caricat. sur Chine et de nombr. grav. s. bois. gr. in-4to. d. veau. 18.—

133a. — **Pontos nos ii, Os.** Lisboa, 1885–5 de fevr. 1891. 7 years in 6
vols. fol. cloth. 60.—
    Principally a political-satirical periodical, criticizing the events in the in-
    terior as well as in foreign countries. It may be considered as a continuation
    to ,,António Maria".
    All published.

134. **Caricatures, Satyre. — Psst ...!** Images par Forain, Caran d'Ache.
Paris, 1898–99. Nos. 1–85. — **Sifflet.** (Dessins par H. G. Ibels).
Paris, 1898–99. Year I–II, nos. 1–20 (= 72 nos.). — Bound in 2
vols. fol. Hfcalf.   40.—
      Psst contains caricatures against Dreyfus and his supporters, Sifflet is
      pro-Dreyfus. Both sets are combined in one chronological order and both
      are complete.

135. — **Rire, Le.** Paris, 1894–1931. T. 1–37. 37 vol. Av. ill. en couleurs
p. Forain, Caran d'Ache, Léandre, Willette, Jossot, Veber, Paw-
lowski, e.a. 4to. d. rel.   275.—
      Un des meilleures périodiques satiriques, illustrés par des artistes de
      premier rang.
      Il ne manque que le no. 33 de l'année 25.

136. — **Sibenicky.** Praze, 1919, 20. Année II, nos. 1 (mai) – 50. Av. ill.
en couleurs. fol. En nos.   7.50
      Feuille satyrique dans le genre du „Simplicissimus".

137. — **Simplicissimus.** Illustrierte Wochenschrift. München, 1896–1934.
Year 1–38. 66 vols. fol. orig. cloth. *Fine copy.*   325.—
      The best satirical weekly for years, published in Germany.

138. — **Smich republiky.** Le rire de la république. Praze, 1919, 20. Année
I, nos. 2–42, 43, II, nos. 1–13. Av. ill en couleurs. gr. in-4to. En
nos.   15.—
      Journal satyrique et humoristique. Année I, no. 1 manque.

139. — **Trombinoscope, Le,** par Touchatout. Dessins (portraits caricatures gravés sur bois) de G. Lafosse. (Paris, 1871–73). Nos. 1 à 83.
En 1 vol. d. rel.   5.—
      Les nos. 10–12, 18 et 39–41 manquent.

140. — **Alhoy, M., y L. Huart,** Los ciento uno Roberto Macario. Escr.
en Frances. Mexico, 1860. Chap. I–L. W. 50 pl. after Daumier.
Hfcalf.   24.—

141. — **Blum, A.,** [Collection d'ouvrages et écrits sur la caricature en
France]. Paris, 1910–21. 10 vol. et pièces. Av. de nombr. ill. 4to et
8vo.   24.—
      L'estampe satirique en France pendant les guerres de religion. — L'es-
      tampe satirique et la caricature en France au 18e siècle. — La caricature
      révolutionnaire. — La caricature en France sous le Directoire et sous
      le Consulat et l'Empire. (2 pièces. Extr.). — La caricature polit. sous la
      monarchie de juillet. — La caricature polit. en France sous le Second Em-
      pire, sous la seconde République et pendant la guerre de 1870–1871. (3
      pièces, dont 2 extr.). — La caricature de guerre en France et à l'étranger.

142. — **Champfleury,** Histoire de la caricature. Paris, 1867–85. 5 vol.
Av. 500 ill. d. rel. Bradel, non rogné, couv. cons.   15.—
      I. Caricature antique. — II. Moyen-âge et sous la Renaissance. — III.
      Sous la Réforme et la Ligue. — Louis XIII à Louis XVI. — IV. Sous la
      République, l'Empire et la Restauration. — V. Caricature moderne.

143. — — Le musée secret de la caricature. Paris, 1888. Av. 69. ill.
d. rel. Bradel, non rogné, couv. cons.   3.50
      Contient e.a.: Caraqueuz en Turquie. — Fêtes et divertissements des tri-
      bus Arabes dans les camps. — La danse des morts au Japon. — Prover-
      bes japonais. — Kruptadia. — etc.

144. — **Fuchs, E.,** Ein vormärzliches Tanzidyll. Lola Montez in der
Karikatur. Berlin, no. d. W. pl. and ill. cloth.   3.—

145. — **Furniss, H.,** The confessions of a caricaturist. London, 1901.
2 vols. W. numer. pl. and ill. cloth.   12.—

Prices are in guilders

146. **Caricatures, Satyre. — Gaudy, F.,** Das Karikaturenbuch. Hrsg.
    von F. von Zobeltitz. Verklein. Ausg. Berlin, 1906. W. 61 pl.
    square-fol.   1.50

147. **— Jacob, De ware.** Weekblad voor scherts en luim, onder leiding
    van J. H. Speenhoff. Rott. 1901–15. Year 1–10. 11 vols. W. numer.
    pl. and ill. by Kees van Dongen, Willy Sluiter, Speenhoff a.o. fol.
    bound.   60.—
    One of the best Dutch satyrical periodicals.

148. **— Juynboll, W. R.,** Het komische genre in de Italiaansche schilder-
    kunst gedur. de 17e en de 18e eeuw. Bijdr. tot de geschiedenis van
    de caricatuur. Leiden, 1934.   3.50

149. **— Kursell, O. von,** Revolutionäre Zeitgenossen. München, 1919.
    2 parts contain. 40 caricatures of Ebert, Liebknecht, Ledebour,
    Eisner, Lenin, Rosa Luxemburg, Erzberger, a.o. roy.4to. In orig.
    cover.   3.—

150. **— Kijker, De.** Geïllustreerd, humoristisch, satyriek weekblad voor
    tooneel, muziek, politiek, enz. Amst. 1899–1902. 3 years (= 88 nos.).
    W. pl. and ill. fol. and roy. 4to. In 1 vol. bound.   20.—
    Satyrical periodical for the greater part devoted to music and the
    theatre.
    All published.

151. **— Musée** des hommes du siècle. Brux. (1891). 24 portr. caricat.
    en couleurs. gr. in-fol. toile.   4.—
    Auteurs. — Princes. — Musiciens. — Savants. — etc.

152. **— Ortego, F.,** Recueil de caricatures. Collection of caricatures.
    Madrid, (ab. 1850). 12 series each of 16 pl. Tog. 192 lithographs,
    with spanish titles. In 1 vol. square 4to. cloth.   20.—

153. **— Paljas.** Geïllustreerd weekblad gewijd aan kunst, humor en
    satire. Onder red. van Ton van Tast. Amst. 1911. 39 nos. W. numer.
    pl. and ill. (some in colours) by Jordaan, Ton van Tast, a.o. fol.
    In 1 vol. hfcloth.   25.—
    Interesting satyrical periodical on Dutch politics, literature etc. Very
    scarce.

154. **— Pinheiro, R. Bordallo,** Album do caricatures phrases e anexins
    da lingua portugueza. Pref. p. J. C. Machado. Lisboa, 1876. W. 10
    pl. square 4to.   4.—

155. **— Raemaekers, L.,** Twintig opnamen uit mijn carico-plane. Amst.
    1910. 20 political caricatures in colours (Th. Heemskerk, A. Kuyper,
    S. van Houten, H. L. Drucker, P. J. Troelstra a.o.). roy. 4to. —
    L. J. Jordaan en **W. F. Winter,** Binnenlandsche politiek en buiten-
    landsche gebeurtenissen. 1911–1913. Amst. 1913. 56 political pl.
    square 4to.   4.—

156. **Carrier-pigeons. — Spruyt, C. A. M.,** De postduivenrassen. Vol-
    ledige beschrijving van alle rassen, met uitvoerigen standaard.
    Gouda, 1938. W. 104 ill. cloth.   4.—

157. **Celts. — Congrès celtique internat.** Saint-Brieuc 1867. Séances,
    Mémoires. Annexes. Saint-Brieuc, 1868. 2 vol.   12.50
    Publication de la Société d'émulation des Côtes-du-Nord.

158. **— Monumenta** historica Celtica. Notices of the Celts in the writings
    of the Greek and Latin authors from the 10th century b. C.
    to the 5th century. Arranged chronolog. w. translation, comment-

ary, glossary, etc. by W. Dinan. London, 1911. T. I (seul). toile.
(9.—)   4.50
> Hecataeus of Miletus. — Himilco. — Pytheas. — Polybius. — etc.

159. **Celts. — Pelloutier, S.**, Histoire des Celtes, et particul. des Gaulois
et des Germains, depuis les temps fabuleux, jusqu'à la prise de
Rome par les Gaulois. La Haye, 1750. 2 vol.   3.—

160. **— Revue celtique.** Publ. avec le concours des principaux savants
des îles Britanniques et du continent. Paris, 1870–1929. T. 1–46.
46 vol., dont 31 d. veau, le reste en livr.   825.—

161. **China. — Adam, M.**, Us et coutumes de la région de Péking d'après
le Je Sia Kieou Wen K'ao, ch. 146–148. Pékin, 1930. Av. 8 pl. 4to.
                                                 8.50

162. **— Chavannes, E.**, Le T'ai Chan. Essai de monographie d'un culte
chinois. Paris, 1910. Av. plan et 61 pl. et ill. *Epuisé*.   20.—
> Annales du Musée Guimet. Bibliothèque d'étude. T. 21.

163. **— Histoire générale** de la Chine ou annales de cet empire. Trad. du
Tong-Kien-Kang Mou p. J. A. M. de Moyriac de Mailla. Publ. p.
Grosier. Paris, 1777–85. 13 vols. W. maps and pl. and atlas of 65
maps and pl. Tog. 14 vols. 4to. fawn-coloured calf, gilt edges. 200.—
> Fine, complete copy, with the rare last two vols., in a contemporary
> binding.

164. **— Kircher S. J., A.**, China monumentis qua sacris qua profanis,
nec non variis naturae et artis spectaculis ill. Amst., J. Janssonius
à Waesberghe, 1667. Av. front., portr., carte, pl. et ill. dans le texte.
fol. veau fleurdelisé. (Rel. fatiguée).   30.—
> Livre singulier. Il est le premier livre ou l'on trouve gravé les caractères
> de l'alphabet Devangacy.

165. **— Laò-Tsé**, Taòte king. A. d. Chines., eingel. und comment. von
V. von Strauss. Lpz. 1870. d. rel.   15.—
> Impression originale, rare. Nom sur le titre.

166. **— —** Même ouvrage. A. d. Chines. von R. von Plaenckner. Lpz.
1870. d. veau.   6.—

167. **— Martini, M.**, Historie van den Tartarschen oorloch, in dewelcke
wert verhaelt, hoe de Tartaren in dese onse eeuw in 't Sineesche
Rijck syn gevallen. U. h. Lat. Utrecht, G. Nieuwenhuysen, (ab.
1670). W. map and 8 pl. sm. 8vo. vellum. (Binding damaged). 15.—

168. **— Mély, F. de**, De Périgueux au Fleuve Jaune. Paris, 1927. Av.
carte et 20 pl. d'objets d'art. 4to.   2.—

169. **— Prip-Møller, J.**, Chinese Buddhist monasteries. Their plan and
its function as a setting for Buddhist monastic life. Copenhague,
1937. W. front. in colours, 4 large folding plans and 365 reprod.,
several at full-page size. fol. Hfvellum.   60.—
> The author is a danish architect, who lived from 1921–1933 in China
> and traveled through this country from North to South and from the East
> up to the Tibetian frontier. The first two chapters give an analysis of the
> construction and division of the Buddhist monastery, according to its
> present aspect, with retrospect to the past; the following two chap. treat
> of the architectural history of the famous monastery Pao Hua Shan;
> the last two deal with the history and daily life of the order of the Buddhist
> monks.

170. **— Thomas, J. A.**, A pioneer tobacco merchant in the Orient.
Durham, 1928. W. 12 pl. cloth. (9.60)   3.—
> The author tells his personal experiences as a tobacco merchant in China.

171. **China. — Treat, P. J.,** The Far East. Political and diplomatic history. N. York, 1928. W. 14 maps. cloth. (9.60) 3.50

172. **— Woodhead, H. G. W.,** The Yangtsze and its problems. Shanghai, 1931. cloth. (4.50) 2.—

173. **— Zeitschrift, Ostasiatische.** Berlin, 1912–34. Year 1–20. 20 vols. in 19. W. numer. maps. pl. and ill. 4to. Hfcloth. 675.—
Very important especially for the fine arts of the Far East. Extremely scarce.

174. **Colonies, Colonisation. — (Becher, J. J.),** Gründlicher Bericht von Beschaffenheit und Eigenschafft, Cultivirung und Bewohnung dess in America zwischen dem Rio Orinoque und Rio de las Amazones .... in Guinea gelegenen Strich Landes, welche die Westindische Compagnie an Friederich Casimir, Grafen zu Hanaw den 18. Julii 1669 überlassen hat. Franckfurt, 1670. W. folding map, meas. 40×35 cM., engraved by J. P. Thelott, 1669. 4to. calf. (44 pp.). 450.—
Not mentioned by Sabin. E x c e s s i v e l y r a r e b o o k l e t, e s-p e c i a l l y w i t h t h e m a p.
The scope of this work was to make propaganda for founding a German colony on the territory between the Orinoco and Amazonas. The author, Becher, was the first to promote this enterprise and on his instigation Count Frederic Casimir of Hanau was in 1669 invested by the Dutch West India Company with this territory extending over 3000 square miles. The author gives first details of the reason for having printed his book, and then treats the methods to be employed in the cultivation of the land, the privileges, etc.

175. **— Beschrijvinge, Pertinente,** van Guiana. Gelegen aen de vaste kust van America. Waer in .... het aenmerckelijkste dat in en omtrent het landt van Guiana valt, als de limiten, het klimaet en de stoffen der landen, de mineralen...., vruchten, dieren ..... Als oock de conditien van de Staten van Hollandt, voor die gene die nae Guiana begeeren te varen. Amst., J. C. ten Hoorn, 1676. W. wood-cut on titlepage and a map. 4to. vellum. 225.—
„Accurate description of Guiana situated on the coast of America. With addition of the profits of the share holders and the conditions for those who wish to sail for Guiana".
A very interesting item containing the conditions granted by the States of Holland to all willing to found a colony on the coast of America.

176. **— Bulletin de la Société d'études coloniales.** Réd. L. Wodon, R. Vauthier e.a. Brux. 1894–1925. Année I–XXXII. Ens. 28 vol. Av. cartes et pl. dont 22 vol. d. rel., le reste en livr. 225.—

177. **— Chéradame, A.,** La colonisation et les colonies allemandes. Paris, 1905. Av. 8 cartes en couleurs se dépliant. d. veau, tête dor. *Bel ex.* 7.50
La fondation des colonies allemandes. — De la condition juridique des colonies. — Description des colonies. Exposé de leur organisation adminis-trative et de leur développement économique.

178. **— Congo.** Revue générale de la colonie belge. Dir. V. Denyn et E. de Jonghe. Brux. 1920–38. Année 1–19. 19 vol. Av. qq. pl. et figg. Av. table des années 1–6. En livr. (190.—) 120.—
Cette revue donne un nombre d'articles intéressants tant sur la géogra-phie, l'ethnologie, le folk-lore, l'histoire naturelle que sur les relations com-merciales, la statistique et la politique de cette partie de l'Afrique Occiden-tale qui forme le règne colonial belge. Elle contient des contributions de L. Franck, V. H. van den Plas, E. de Wildeman, R. Caluwaert, e.a.

179. **Colonies. — Congrès internat. colonial, 14e.** Bruxelles 1897. Compte
rendu. Brux. 1897.   6.—
180. — — Idem. Paris 1900. Rapports, mémoires et procès-verbaux.
(Paris), 1901.   5.—
181. — — Idem, 3e. Gand 1913. Compte rendu. Gand, 1922. 2 vol. 9.—
182. — **Congrès colonial.** Marseille 1906. Compte rendu des travaux.
Paris, 1907, 08. T 1, II, IV. 3 vol.   7.50
183. — **Congrès colonial français.** Paris 1907. Paris 1908.   3.50
184. — **Congrès colonial national.** Paris 1889–1890. Recueil des déli-
bérations. Paris, 1890, 92. 3 vol., dont 2. d. veau, 1 br.   6.—
185. — — Idem, 3e. Bruxelles 1930. Rapports. Comptes rendus. Brux.
1930, 31. 2 vol.   4.50
186. — **Congresso, 1ro,** di studi coloniali. Firenze 1931. Atti. Firenze,
1932–33. 7 vol. Av. qq. pl.   35.—
187. — — Idem, 2°. Napoli 1934. Atti. Firenze, 1936–37. 7 vol. 35.—
188. — — Idem, 3°. Atti. Firenze, 1937. 9 vol. Av. qq. pl.   35.—
189. — **Congrès** de la colonisation. Montreal 1898. Rapport. Montreal,
1900.   3.—
190. — **(Dessalles, P.**), Annales du conseil souverain de la Martinique,
ou tableau histor. du gouvernement de cette colonie . . . . auquel
on a joint l'analyse raisonnée des loix qu'y ont été publiées. Berge-
rac, 1786. 2 vol. 4to. vél. vert.   225.—
        Ouvrage monumental, remarquablement documenté, et qui est la source
        fondamentale pour l'histoire de cette colonie et par la même occasion de
        l'histoire de la colonisation française dans les Antilles. Les documents
        qui y sont reproduits ont été détruits.
        De la plus grande rareté.
191. — **Grol, G. J. van,** De grondpolitiek in het Westindische domein der
Generaliteit. I. Algemeen histor. inleiding. 's-Grav. 1934. cloth. 2.—
192. — **H(erlein), J. D.,** Beschryvinge van de volk-plantinge Zuriname,
vertonende de opkomst dier zelver colonie, de aanbouw en bewer-
kinge der zuiker-plantagien, den aard der Indianen, als ook de
slaafsche Afrikaansche mooren. . . . de bosch-grond, water- en
pluymgedierten, vrugten, gommen, olyen en de gesteltheit van de
Karaïbaansche kust. Leeuwarden, M. Injema, 1718. W. front.,
map and pl. 4to. Hfvellum. *Very tall copy.*   60.—
        Pp. 249–262: Karaïbaansch woordenboek.
193. — **Jahresbericht** über die Entwicklung der deutschen Schutzge-
biete 1896–97–1901/02. Berlin, 1898–1903. 6 vol. Av. cartes. 4to.
d. rel.   30.—
        Beilage zum Deutschen Kolonialblatt.
193a. — **Kat Angelino, A. D. A. de,** Colonial policy. Abridged transl.
from the Dutch by G. J. Renier in collabor. with the author.
The Hague, 1931. 2 vols. cloth. (18.—)   12.—
        I. General principles. — II. The Dutch East Indies.
194. — **Keye, O.,** Kurtzer Entwurff von Neu-Niederland und Guajana
einander entgegen gesetzt, umb den Unterschied zwischen warmen
und kalten Landen herausz zu bringen, und zu weisen welche von
beyden am füglichsten zu bewohnen, ... Denen Patronen, so da
Colonien an zu legen gesonnen . . . . A. d. Holländ. d. T. R. C. S. C.
S. (Th. Ritsch). Lpz. 1672. 4to. boards.   325.—
        Asher no. 12. The German edition also is of great rarity.

Prices are in guilders

195. **Colonies. — Kongo-Overzee.** Tijdschrift voor en over Belgisch Kongo, Ruanda-Urundi en aanpalende gewesten. Onder red. van A. Burssens. Antw. 1934–38. Année I–IV. 4 vol. Av. ill. En livr. 24.—
Ce périodique, paraissant tous les deux mois, contient des contributions sur l'ethnographie, la linguistique, la mission, l'art indigène, l'histoire coloniale, le droit des indigènes, etc. du Congo belge et des régions voisines.

196. **— Labernadie, M. V.,** Le vieux Pondichéry. 1673–1815. Histoire d'une ville coloniale française. Av. préf. de A. Martineau. Pondichéry, 1936. Av. 3 plans et 10 pl.   5.—

197. **— Mittheilungen von Forschungsreisenden und Gelehrten aus den deutschen Schutzgebieten** (later: Mitteilungen aus den deutschen Schutzgebieten). Hrsg. von Von Danckelmann, u. A. Berlin, 1888–1930.36 vols. 4to and 8vo. W. „Ergänzungshefte". 16 vols. 4to. — Tog. 52 vols. W. numer. large maps, pl. and ill. 19 vols. hfcalf, the remainder in parts.   475.—
E x t r e m e l y s c a r c e a n d m u c h s o u g h t a f t e r. Complete sets are hardly available. These volumes were published as „Beihefte zum deutschen Kolonialblatt".

198. **— Organisation** politique et administrative des colonies. Brux. 1936.   7.80
Contient: **M. Halewyck de Heusch,** Les institutions politiques et administratives des pays africains soumis à l'autorité de la Belgique. **— A. Malvezzi de Medici,** Organisation politique et administrative des colonies italiennes. **— Ph. Kleintjes,** Institutions politiques et administratives des pays d'outremer néerlandais. — etc.
Publ. par la Bibliothèque coloniale internat.

199. **— Pecci Contreras, M.,** y **L. de Madariaga y de la Torre,** Il imperio aleman colonial. Madrid, 1918. W. map.   1.50

200. **— Plante Fébure, J. M.,** West-Indië in het Parlement, 1897–1917. Bijdrage tot Nederlands koloniaal-politieke geschiedenis. 's-Grav. 1918. (5.40)   2.—

201. **— Pyttersen, Tj.,** Een deel der taak van Nederland in Suriname. 's-Grav. 1927.   1.20

202. **— —** Europeesche kolonisatie in Suriname. Geschiedkund. schets. 's-Grav. 1896.   1.—

203. **— Raders, R. F. van,** Geschiedkund. aanteek. rakende proeven van Europeesche kolonisatie in Suriname. 's-Grav. 1860. Av. carte. toile.   4.—

204. **— Revue indigène, La.** Organe des intérêts des indigènes aux colonies et pays de protectorat. Paris, 1906–19, 22. Année 1–14, 17 (= nos. 1–132, 157–168). Rel. en 10 vol. d. veau.   58.—
„La Revue indigène se fonde pour apporter son concours aux bonnes volontés qui cherchent à relever la condition de l'indigène".

205. **— Robin, C. C.,** Voyages dans l'intérieur de la Louisiane, de la Floride occidentale, et dans les isles de la Martinique et de Saint-Domingue pendant les années 1802–1806. Conten. de nouv. observat. sur l'histoire naturelle, les moeurs, le commerce, les maladies, partic. le fièvre jaune. En outre ce qui s'est passé rel. à l'établissement des Anglo-Américains en Louisiane. Suiv. de la flore Louisianaise. Paris, 1807. 3 vol. Av. portrait et carte se dépliant, gravée en couleurs. veau.   65.—

206. **Colonies. — Teenstra,. M. D.**, De negerslaven in de kolonie Suriname. Dordrecht, 1842. Av. carte et 1 pl. lithogr., représent. e.a.
l'incendie de Paramaribo. cart. orig.   6.—
Les pp. 1—79 traitent de la colonie, de son agriculture, et de sa popula-
tion (libre), les pp. 177–308 de l'incendie de Paramaribo (1832) et de
l'exécution de 3 nègres, les pp. 311—380 contiennent une bibliographie
raisonnée.

207. **— Verlaine, L.**, Notre colonie. Contrib. à la recherche de la méthode
de colonisation. Brux. 1923. 2 vol.   1.50
I. La méthode d'évaluation des virtualités individuelles et sociales des
nègres. — II. La méthode de colonisation.

208. **— Vestiging, De**, van de Nederlandsche kolonisten in Suriname
herdacht, 1845–1870. Paramaribo, 1921. Av. 1 pl.   1.—

209. **Conclave. — Pianta, Nuova e esatta**, del Conclave con le funtioni e
ceremonie per l'elettione del nuovo Pontefice, fatto nella sede va-
cante di Papa Innocenti XII, nel quale entrorno l'em. sig. cardinali
adi IX di Ottobre 1700. Roma, D. Rossi, 1700. Av. 7 pl. fol. vél.
                                                            25.—
Dans la même reliure 14 vues de la ville de Rome, la Sicile, etc. p. Rossi
et Specchi.

210. **Couperus, L.**, Eline Vere. Een Haagsche roman. Amst. 1889. 3 vol.
d. rel.   15.—
Première édition, fort rare.

211. **— Wereldvrede.** Amst. 1895.   3.50
Edition originale.

212. **Crusius, Chr. A.**, Gründliche Belehrung vom Aberglauben. A. d.
Lat. von C. F. Pezold. Lpz. 1767. d. veau.   6.—

213. **Danube. — Marsili, A. F.**, Danubius Pannonico-mysicus, observa-
tionibus geographicis, astronomicis, hydrographicis, historicis,
physicis perlustratus. Hag. Com., P. Gosse, R. Chr. Alberts, P.
de Hondt, Amst., H. Uytwerf, et F. Changuion, 1726. 6 vols.
W. 6 front. by Houbraken and Ottens, 282 maps and pl., illustr.
of the scenery, natural history, antiquities, etc. connected with
the Danube and numer. remarkable vign., culs-de-lampe and
initials. imp. fol. Hfvellum. *Large paper copy.*   225.—
A complete copy of this remarkable and magnificent work is very rare.

214. **Danzig. — Malcomess, H.**, Der Erwerb und Verlust der Danziger
Staatsangehörigkeit auf Grund des Gesetzes vom 30 Mai 1922.
Ihlau, 1932.   1.50

214*a*. **— Prinzhorn, F.**, Danzig-Polen-Korridor und Grenzgebiete.
Bibliographie mit besond. Berücksicht. von Politik und Wirt-
schaft, 1931 und 1932. Danzig, 1932, 33. Année I. pet. in-fol.
En livr. (25.—)   15.—

215. **Diezel, G.**, Deutschland und die abendländische Civilisation. Stuttgart, 1852. **— Id.**, Die Frage der deutschen Zukunft. Stuttgart,
1854. **— Id.**, Russland, Deutschland und die östliche Frage. Stuttgart, 1853. **— En 1 vol. d. veau.**   15.—
Le premier ouvrage fut défendu.

216. **(Drost, A.)**, Schetsen en verhalen. Amst. 1835, 36. 1 tom. 2 vol. Av.
titre lith. et portr.   10 —
Contient e.a.: De pestilentie te Katwijk.

217. **Eden, F. van**, Enkele verzen. Amst. 1898. *Orig. cover.*   7.50
Fine copy of the original edition.

                        Prices are in guilders

218. **Epitaphs. — Grafschriften** in Stad en Lande. Verz. en uitgeg. d. J. A. Feith, C. H. van Rijn, J. Vinhuizen en G. A. Wumkes. Groningen, 1910. W. 19 pl. and numer. heraldic figg. cloth. *Out of print.* 20.—

219. **Fascism. — Annuaire** (du) Centre international d'études sur le fascisme (Cinef). La Haye, 1928–30. 3 vol.   7.50
Le Cinef, groupement entièrement indépendant, fondé à Lausanne en 1927, a pour but l'étude objective et scientifique du fascisme et des mouvements analogues.
Tout ce qui a paru.

220. **Georgisch, P.**, Regesta chronologico-diplomatica, in quibus recesentur omnis generis monumenta et documenta publica [305–1730]. Francof. 1740–44. 4 vols. in 2. fol. vellum.   45.—
Important work, containing a catalogue of all the printed diplomatic documents.

221. **Greenland. —Atuagagdliutit** nalínginarnik tusaruminásassumik univkát, 1861–1936/37. Godthaab, 1861–1937. W. numer. maps and pl., coloured and plain. 4to. Partly bound, uncut, or in the original parts.   600.—
The only periodical printed in Greenland; of the greatest importance for the study of history, ethnography, etc. of the Eskimos. Part of the text is written by Eskimos and many of the plates are executed after designs made by Eskimos.
Extremely rare in complete state.

222. **Gretna Green. — Hutchinson, P. O.**, De kronyk van Gretna Green. N. h. Eng. Deventer, 1844. Av. grav. sur le titre. cart. orig., n.r.   5.—
Bel ex. en cartonnage original, ill. d'une gravure avec inscription: Hier trouwt men de lieden.
Marque de bibliothèque sur le titre.

223. **Hafed, Prince of Persia.** Experiences in earth-life and spirit-life. Spirit communications received through D. Duguid. W. append. contain. Communications from Ruisdal and Steen. London, 1876. Av. pl. toile.   3.50

224. **Haller, C. L. von,** Restauration der Staats-Wissenschaft oder Theorie des natürlich-geselligen Zustands der Chimäre des künstlich-bürgerlichen entgegengesetzt. 2e verm. Aufl. Winterthur, 1820–34. 6 vols. W. lith. portrait. Hfcalf.   60.—
I. Darstellung, Geschichte und Critik der bisherigen falschen Systeme (519 pp.). — II. Von den Fürstenthümern oder Monarchien. Von den unabhängigen Grundherren. (602 pp.). — III. Makrobiotik der Patrimonial-Staaten. Von den unabhängigen Feldherren. (594 pp.). — IV. Von den unabhängigen geistlichen Herren oder den Priester-Staaten. (447 pp.). — V. Makrobiotik der geistlichen Herrschaften oder Priester-Staaten. (376 pp.). — VI. Von den Republiken oder freyen Communitäten. (596 pp.).
„Haller steht vor uns als ein Mann von gewaltiger Kraft des Geistes . . . . er hat ein Werk geliefert, welches seinen Namen auf die späte Nachwelt bringen wird". (Mohl).
Very scarce, especially with the 5th vol. which is often wanting.

225. **Hanfstaengl, E. F. S.**, Amerika und Europa von Marlborough bis Mirabeau. München, 1930. W. 3 maps and 38 pl. bound. (9.—) 4.50

226. **Hinrichs, H. F. W.**, Die Könige. Entwicklungsgeschichte des Königtums von den ältesten Zeiten bis auf die Gegenwart. Lpz. 1852.   5.—
Les derniers ff. tachés d'eau.

227. **Hitler, A.,** Mon combat. Traduction intégrale de „Mein Kampf" par J. Gaudefroy-Demombynes et A. Calmettes. Paris, (1934). sewed, uncut.   25.—
     Perfect copy in new condition of the original edition, made after the f i r s t german edition, of the french translation. Withdrawn by the publishers and never put on the market.

228. **House of Orange: William the Silent.** — Apologie ou défense de tresillustre prince Guillaume .... prince d'Orange .... contre le Ban et edict publié par le Roi d'Espaigne .... Ens. ledict ban ou proscription. (Leyde), Ch. Sylvius, 1581. Av. les armoiries de la Maison d'Orange-Nassau (2×) et la marque de l'imprimeur à la fin. 4to. veau, av. dentelles, dos doré. *Bel ex., grand de marges.* 100.—
     Knuttel, no. 555. Tiele, no. 226. Edition, publ. dans la même année que la première, de la célèbre apologie de Guillaume le Taciturne.

229. — — **Bekentnus** der durchleuchtigesten Fürsten, Wilhelm Printz zu Vranien, sampt andern jrer F. G. Mitverwandten Defension vñ Nothwehr wider des Duca de Alba Vnchristliche unnd vnerhörte verfolgung gegen alle Stendt der Niederlanden. No pl. 1568. 4to. boards.   60.—
     Other edition than Knuttel, no. 167. First German edition of the „Rescript et declaration du.... Prince d'Orange".

230. — — **Beschreibung, Warhafftige und eigentliche,** von der Geburt, Leben und Sterben desz Printzen von Orangien, Graff Wilhelm vonn Nassauw, umbkommen ist. Auch mit was Tormenten, Marter und Pein Balthasar Serack, so die That gethan, derhalben zu Delfft in Hollandt vom leben zum Todt gebracht. Cölln, J. Büchsenmechr, 1584. W. engraving on titlepage, represent. the murder of the prince and the torturing of the murderer. 4to.   45.—
     Knuttel, nr. 696. Very scarce. Different from the edition, described in Fruin, Verspreide geschriften, vol. III.

231. — — **Discours** oft verhael ghemaect op de quetsure van mijn Heere de Prince van Oraignen. No pl. 1582. 4to. Hfvellum.   25.—
     Knuttel, nr. 598.

232. — — **Discours** du meurdre commis en la personne du tres illustre Prince d'Orange. No pl. 1584. 4to.   25.—
     Knuttel, nr. 691.

233. — — **Guillaume le Taciturne,** Correspondance. Publ. p. L. P. Gachard. Brux. 1847–66. 6 vol. buckram. *Epuisé.*   65.—

234. — — **Historie** Balthazars Gerardt, alias Serach, die den tyran van 't Nederlandt den Prince van Orangie doorschoten heeft: ende is daerom duer grouwelijcke ende vele tormenten binnen de stadt van Delft openbaerlijck ghedoodt. No pl. 1584. 4to. boards.   40.—
     Knuttel, No. 693. See for the particulars of this scandalous and infamous pamphlet: Fruin, Verspreide geschriften III, 87 etc.
     Extremely scarce. Titlepage waterstained.

235. — — **Justification, La,** du Prince d'Oranges, contre les faulx blasmes, que ses calumniateurs taschent à luy imposer à tort. No pl., Imprimé au moys d'Apuril 1568. sm. 8vo. vellum, gilt edges. (Mod. binding). *Fine, tall copy.*   100.—
     Knuttel, nr. 159. Tiele, nr. 82. This french original is very scarce. The pamphlet is attributed to H. Languet. See: Archives de la Maison d'Orange-Nassau, III, p. 186.

236. — — **Moord, De,** van 1584. Oorspronk. verhalen en berichten van den moord op Prins Willem van Oranje. M. bijl. en aanteek. uit-

geg. d. J. G. Frederiks. 's-Grav. 1884. Av. belle eau-forte p. J. P.
Arendsen d'après un dessin, fait pour ce livre p. J. Bosboom. pet.
in-8vo. 7.50
Collection de récits contemporains de l'assassinat de Guillaume I. Imprimé à 325 exx. et épuisé.

238. **House of Orange: William the Silent.** — **Rachfahl, F.**, Wilhelm von Oranie und der Niederland. Aufstand. Halle, Haag, 1906–24. Vol. 1–3 (–1569). 3 vols. cloth. (37.50) 17.—
Standard work on the youth of William the Silent. All published.

239. — — **Recueil, Bref,** de l'assasinat commis en la personne du Prince d'Orange, Comte de Nassau, etc. par Jean Jauregui Espaignol. Suivent les copies des pappiers trouvez sur l'assassinateur; les dépositions des criminels, lettres d'Añastro et du prince de Parme. Anvers, Plantin, 1582. 4to. 40.—
Knuttel, nr. 593.
Slightly waterstained.

240. — — **Remonstrance** faite a Messievrs les depvtez des Estats Generavlx le IXme de januier 1580 par Mons. le Prince d'Oranges. Anvers, Giles vanden Rade, s. d. 4to. 20.—
Knuttel, nr. 523. Le Prince parle des pertes de l'année 1579, dues à l'irrésolution des Néerlanlais: ,,La vraye cause de tant de maux est nostre irresolution, car nous assemblons assez, nous consultons longuement et au contraire sommes aussi negligens à executer comme nous sommes diligens à deliberer". Il démontre la nécessité d'une bonne armée: ,,Je ne voy point comment il est possible de faire teste à l'ennemy.... si non que nous ayons un corps d'armee composé pour le moins de quatre mille cheuaulx et douze mil hommes de pied".

241. — — **Verantwoordinge, De,** des Princen van Orangien, tegen de valsche logenen, daer mede sijn wedersprekers hem soecken tonrechte te beschuldighen. No pl. 1569. sm. 8vo. vellum. 75.—
Other edition than Knuttel, no. 160. This pamphlet has been attributed to H. Languet.
See: Archives de la Maison d'Orange-Nassau, III, p. 186. The french original appeared in 1568.

242. — — **Verhael, Cort,** van 't moordadich feyt geperpetreert inden persoone van den Prince van Oraengien, Graue van Nassau, etc. by Jan Jauregui Spaengnaert. Antw., Chr. Plantijn, 1582. 4to. hfvellum. (Mod. binding). 75.—
Knuttel, nr. 590. Account of the attempt on the life of William the Silent by Jean Jauregui, 1582. With a large number of letters a.o. offic. documents, several of which in spanish. Very scarce.

243. — — **Verhael, Cort,** van de moort, ghedaen aen den persoone van den Prince van Orangien. (Antw.) 1584. W. 2 pl. added. 40.—
Knuttel, nr. 690. Official account of the murder of William the Silent, written by order of the States-General. Most of the later historians have based their descriptions on it. The text is the same as that of the original edition. (Knuttel, nr. 688).
,,The basis of this account was the confession of Balthazar, written in the convent of Saint Agatha.... immediately after his arrest, together with his answers to the interrogatories between the 10th and 14th July. (Motley, The rise, etc. III, 599).

244. — — **Verklaers** ende wtschrift des .... heeren Willem, Prince van Orangien etc. ende zijner Excellentien nootsakelicke defensie teghen den Duca de Alba, ende zijne grouwelijcke tyrannye. S. l. (1568). 4to. 50.—
Van der Wulp, no. 189. Autre édition chez Tiele, no. 79. Pas chez Knuttel.

Mart. Nijhoff, The Hague — Cat. No. 630

Bor, I, 254. Justification de Guillaume le Taciturne écrite sur son instigation contre le duc d'Albe, et en même temps pour encourager les Hollandais.
Bel ex., non rogné, av. le dernier f. blanc.

245. **House of Orange: William the Silent. — Willem I, Prins van
Oranje,** Correspondentie. Uitgeg. d. N. Japikse. 's-Grav. 1934. T. I
(1551–1561). toile.   7.50
Cette publication forme un complément aux publications de Groen van
Prinsterer, ,,Archives ou correspondance inédite de la Maison d'Orange-
Nassau" et de Gachard, ,,Correspondance de Guillaume le Taciturne".
La plupart des lettres du t. I sont en français ou en allemand.
Uitgaven vanwege het Koninklijk Huis-archief. Uitgeg. onder de leiding
van N. Japikse. III.

246. **— Delaborde, J.,** Charlotte de Bourbon, princesse d'Orange.
Paris, 1888. *Epuisé.*   5.—

247. **— —** Louise de Coligny, Princesse d'Orange. Paris, 1890. 2 vol.
Av. 2 portr. d. chagr. rouge.   10.—

248. **— Louise de Coligny,** Lettres à sa belle-file Charlotte-Brabantine
de Nassau, Duchesse de la Trémoille. Publ. d'après les origin. p.
P. Marchegay. Paris, 1872.   3.—

249. **Ibsen, H. — Meir, G.,** De dood en doodssymboliek in Ibsens werken.
Antw. 1938.   8.—
Werken uitgeg. d. de faculteit van de wijsbegeerte en letteren (der)
Rijksuniversiteit te Gent. 84e Afl.

250. **Ireland. — Pressensé, F. de,** L'Irlande et l'Angleterre, depuis l'acte
d'union jusqu'à nos jours, 1800–88. Paris, 1889.   2.50

251. **— Schultze-Hamburg, E.,** Irland. Seine polit. Knechtung und sein
Streben nach Selbst-regierung. Berlin, (1918). W. pl. and portr.
cloth.   2.50

252. **Iron masque, Man with the. — St. Mihiel, De,** Le véritable homme
dit au masque de fer. Strasburg, 1790. d. veau.   3.—

253. **Jansenists. — Bennink Janssonius, R.,** De Jansenistae historia et
principe. Groningae, 1841.   1.—

254. **— Exposition** de la doctrine de l'église Jansénienne, tirée des ré-
flexions morales du P. Quesnel, et des principaux docteurs du
Parti. No pl. 1739. calf.   2.50

255. **— Gerth van Wijk Jr., J. A.,** Historia ecclesiae Ultrajectinae Rom.-
Cath., male Jansenisticae dictae. Ultr. 1859.   1.75

256. **— Hoynck van Papendrecht, K. P.,** Historie der Utrechtsche kerke,
zedert den tyd der veranderde godsdienst in de Vereen. Nederlanden. U. h. Lat. Mechelen, L. van der Elst, 1728. gr. in-fol. d. rel. 5.—

256a. **— Nouvelles ecclésiastiques** ou Mémoires pour servir à l'histoire
de la constitution Unigenitus. Paris, Utrecht, G. vander Weyde,
J. F. Rosart, J. Schelling et P. Muntendam, etc. 1713–1803. 92
années en 21 vol. Av. tables. 3 vol. Ens. 24 vol. Av. front. et grav.
4to. veau.   *Sold*
,,De tous les journaux prohibés aucun ne fit autant de bruit que cette
feuille. La valeur et l'intérêt historiques n'ont pas besoin d'être démontrés;
c'est dans ce recueil qu'on apprend cette longue querelle qui agita la
France pendant le 18e siècle. Les Nouvelles ecclésiastiques s'imprimaient
partout; aujourd'hui dans une ville, demain dans quelque village, dans
une cave ou dans un grenier et jusqu'au fond des bois". (*Hatin*).

Prices are in guilders

Voyez aussi Hatin, p. 57: „La collection la plus complète que je connaisse, se compose de 71 vol., allant de 1728 à 1798".
Dans les années 1771 à 1787, une soixantaine de feuillets est manuscrite en copie de l'époque. Les années 1765, 1766, 1792 et 1793 sont en double (en partie de différentes impressions).
Collection absolument complète, avec les tables, pour ainsi dire introuvable.

257. **Jansenists. — Ritschl, A.,** Die Entstehung der altkatholischen Kirche. 2e (letzte) Aufl. Bonn, 1857. d. veau. 10.—

258. **— Vlaming, P.,** De drie hoofdgeschillen tusschen de Rooms-Catholyken. Wegens I. Formulier tegen Jansenius. II. De bulle Unigenitus. III. Het Aerts-bisdom van Utrecht. Opgehelderd ... tegen een schrift van David Pierman. Utrecht, H. Spruyt, 1739–41. 3 vol. pet. in-8vo. veau. 3.50

259. **Jardine, D.,** The Mad Mullah of Somaliland. London, 1923. W. portrait, 4 maps and 17 pl. cloth. ((9.60) 2.50
The story of the adventurous career of the Mad Mullah from his rise in 1899 to his death in 1920.

260. **Jesuits. — d'Alembert, J.,** Sur la destruction des Jésuites en France. 1765. 9.—
Première édition.

261. **— Boucher, A.,** Histoire dramatique et pittoresque des Jésuites. Paris, (v. 1845). 2 vol. Av. pl., grav. s. acier. d. rel. 4.—

262. **— Cotton, P.,** Brief dienende tot verclaringe vande leere der Vaderen Jesuijten.... Metter Anti-Cotton daer teghen ghestelt. U. h. Fr. 's-Grav. 1610. 4to. 3.50

263. **— Griesinger, Th.,** Die Jesuiten. Vollständ. Geschichte ihrer Wirksamkeit. Stuttgart, 1866. 2 tom. 1 vol. toile. (Dos cassé). 6.—

264. **— Inchofer S. J., M.,** La monarchie des Solipses. Trad. du lat. Amst., H. Uytwerf, 1722. pet. in-8vo. veau. 6.—
La „Monarchia Solipsorum" est un satyre sur l'ordre des Jésuites, dont l'original parut en 1646.
Voyez: Allgem. deutsche Biographie. XIV, 65.

265. **— Jarrigius, P.,** Jesuita in ferali pegmate ob nefanda crimina in provincia Guienna perpetrata. E Gallico latin. donat. Cum judicio generali de hoc Ordine. L. B. 1665. Av. front. 12mo. cart. 18.—
Traduction latine du libelle fameux „Les jésuites mis sur l'échafaud pour plusieurs crimes capitaux", qui parut à Leide en 1648. Voir Willems, Les Elzevier, no. 1655.
Très rare.

266. **— Leutbecher, J.,** Der berühmte Jesuit Juan Maria über den König und dessen Erziehung. Erlangen, 1830. 5.—

267. **— Maronier, J. H.,** De orde der Jezuieten. Geschiedenis, inrichting en moraal. Leiden, 1899. 1.—

268. **— Mémoires, Nouveaux,** des missions de la Compagnie de Jésus, dans le Levant. Paris, 1715–55. 9 vol. Av. 7 cartes se dépliant et 7 pl. pet. in-8vo. veau. 75.—
Les tom. I—VII sont écrits par Th. Ch. Fleurian d'Armenonville, les t. VIII par N. L. Ingoult, le t. IX par A. Roger.
Le t. I est en 2e édition.

269. **— Montgommery, L.,** Le fleau d'Aristogiton. Ou contre le calomniateur des Pères Jésuites, sous le titre d'Anticoton. Av. le re-

merciment des Burieres de Paris. Amst., M. Colyn, 1610. 2 fasc.
5.—

270. **Jesuits.** — **Placaet** van de stadt Bristol in Engeland, door den Prince van Orangien trouppen bezet, inhoud. het verjaegen, en ver-bannen van Jesuiten, priesters, papen, en monnicken.... No pl. 1688. 4to.   12.—
Knuttel, no. 12856.

271. — **Procès des Jésuites.** — **Recueil factice** de 227 opuscules publiés en 1762–1764, rel. à la condamnation et à l'expulsion des Jésuites hors de France. Rel. en 21 vol. pet. in -8vo. veau ancien.   120.—
Très importante collection des documents publiés en France lors du procès des Jésuites devant les divers Parlements et qui se termina par leur condamnation et leur expulsion. On y trouve tous les réquisitoires, plaidoiries, arrêts, extraits des registres de Parlements, relations, et aussi de nombreuses pièces annexes. Le détail de ces pièces s'établit comme suit: Parlement de Paris. 48 ouvrages en 8 vol. — Parlement de Toulouse. 25 ouvrages en 2 vol. — Parlement de Provence. 27 ouvrages en 3 vol. — Bretagne. 20 ouvrages en 1 vol. — Flandre. 5 ouvrages en 1 vol. — Parlement de Normandie. 29 ouvrages en 1 vol. — etc., etc.

272. — **Scott, Th.**, Vox populi.... dienende tot ontdeckinghe van de listige practycquen van de ambitieuse trouloose Spaenjaerden ende de Jesuyten. U. h. Eng. d. J. Hughes. Utrecht, 1625. 4to. d. veau.   6.—

273. — **Sinclair, Cath.**, Beatrice, of de hedendaagsche Jezuiten in Engeland. N. h. Eng. d. C. M. Mensing. Sneek, 1853. 2 vol. Av. titres lith. av. vign.   2.50

274. — **(Weidner, J. L.)**, Jubileum s. speculum Jesuiticum, exhibens praecipua Jesuitarum scelera, molitiones, fraudes, imposturas, et mendacia, contra statum ecclesiasticum, politicumque, in, et extra Europaeum orbem etc. S. l. 1643. 12mo. vél. *Bel ex.*   20.—
Bohemorum de Jesuitis querulae. — Controversiones Indorum quales. — Orbis novus Jesuitarum causa detectus. — Japonicae Epistolae multa narrant, pauca probant. — Japonorum conversiones quales. — Noviomagum patria Canisii. — Puer Japonicus concionator. — Wilhelmus Auraicus Princeps vulneratur. — Danus Sueco bellum debet inferre, sic Jesuitis suadentibus. — Gustavus Adolphus clementer cum Jesuitis agit. — Moscovia à Jesuitis attentata. — Polonia. — Iesuitica societas pedem in Turcico regno ponunt. — etc.

275. — **Wijnmalen, T. C. L.**, Pascal als bestrijder der Jezuiten en ver-dediger des Christendoms. Utrecht, 1865.   3.—

276. — **Zuidema, W.**, De zedeleer der Jezuïeten. Utrecht, 1897. d. rel. (2.25)   1.—

277. **Jouet, A.**, Ce qu'est devenue la victoire. Versailles, Locarno, Genève. Préf. de G. Bouvalot. Paris, 1926.   2.—
Contient e.a.: Les résultats manqués. — La frontière de 1814. — La République Rhénane. — En Savoie. — En Orient. — etc.

278. **Kloos, Willem,** Verzen uit de jaren 1880–1890. 's-Grav. 1919. roy. 8vo. vellum.   60.—
Beautiful work from the famous press ,,De Zilverdistel''. This edition is limited to 120 copies of which only 50 in the trade. Our copy is no. 27. Extremely scarce.

279. **Lindeboom, J.**, Stiefkinderen van het Christendom. 's-Grav. 1929. toile.   10.—
Cet ouvrage contient l'histoire des sectes hérétiques depuis le Manichéisme jusqu'au commencement du 19e siècle.

Prices are in guilders

280. **Mandrake. — Thompson, C. J. S.**, The mystic mandrake. London, 1934. W. 11 pl. and 19 ill. cloth. (9.—) 3.50
   The mandrake (Mandragora) is a very mysterious root which on account of its resemblance to the human form was believed to possess occult properties which could cause it to become animated.

281. **Margaret of Austria. — Kooperberg, L. M. G.**, Margaretha van Oostenrijk, landvoogdes der Nederlanden tot den vrede van Kamerijk (1509). Amst. 1908. Av. portr. (Sans titre). 5.—

282. **— Quinsonas, E. de**, Matériaux pour servir à l'histoire de Marguerite d'Autriche, duchesse de Savoie, regente des Pays-Bas. Paris, 1860. 3 vol. Av. 25 portr. et pl. en couleurs et en noir. 20.—
   I. Histoire et topographie des lieux qu'habita la princesse. — II. Les tombes ducales de Brou et bibliographie (pp. 275–547). — III. Analectes ou choix de pièces justificatives.
   Fort rare.

283. **Marine. — Albion, R. G.**, Square-riggers on schedule. The New Yorck sailing packets te England, France, and the cotton ports. Princeton, 1938. W. portr. and pl. cloth. 7.—

284. **— Bensaude, J.**, Lacunes et surprises de l'histoire des découvertes maritimes. 1e partie (= pp. 255–448) [L'administration coloniale de João II]. Coimbra, 1930. 4to. 6.—
   Pp. 255—302. João II; pp. 303–340: Plan des découvertes portugaises; pp. 341–448: La critique histor. de Camões et la lutte contre l'Islam.
   Les pp. 1–254 probablement n'ont pas été publiées.

285. **— Burchett, J.**, A complete history of the most remarkable transactions at sea, from the earliest accounts of time to the conclusion of the last war with France. Wherein the most considerable naval-expeditions, sea-fights, discoveries,.... partic. of Great Britain from 1688. London, 1720. W. front., portr. by Vertue and 9 charts. fol. calf. (Rebacked). 90.—
   Deals especially with the British history during the reign of William III. Contains also: Of the Swedes, Danes, Muscovites, Turks, etc. Of the naval wars of the Muscovites, and of the Turks. Sir George Rooke's proceedings in the Baltick, for reconciling the Kings of Denmark and Sweden, etc. Laurence Wright sent with a squadron ships to the West Indies (1689) and what happened in those parts during.... his command Capt. Robert Wilmot sent.... to the West Indies, with an account of his proceedings (1694–95). Expedition of Sir Hovenden Walker against Quebec, 1711, etc.

286. **— Deslandes**, Essai sur la marine des anciens et partie. sur leurs vaisseaux de guerre. Paris, 1768. Av. 10 pl. se dépliant. pet. in-8vo. 9.—

287. **— Hennique, P. A.** Une page d'archéologie navale. Les caboteurs et pêcheurs de la côte de Tunisie. Pêche des éponges. Paris, 1888. Av. 63 pl. de différ. types de bateaux. toile orig. 15.—

288. **— Le Roy, D.**, Les navires des anciens, considérés par rapport à leurs voiles, et à l'usage qu'on en pourrait faire dans notre marine. Paris, 1783. Av. 3 grandes pl. veau. 15.—

289. **— Marmol, D. M. M. del**, Idea de los barcos de vapor, ò descripcion de su maquina, relacion de sus progresos, e indicacion de sus ventajas. Sanlucar, 1817. W. 1 pl. sm. 8vo. 18.—

290. **— Seinen, Generale**, voor de Nederl. flotille. 's Grav. 1832. Av. 2 pl. color. de signaux. 5.—

291. **— Sourdis, Henri d'Escoubleau de**, Archevêque de Bordeaux, Correspondance, augm. des ordres et lettres de Louis XIII et du

Cardinal de Richelieu à de Sourdis concern. les opérations des flottes françaises de 1636—1642. Av. texte histor., notes etc. sur l'état de la marine en France, sous Richelieu, p. E. Sue. Paris, 1839. 3 vol. 4to. d. rel., n. r.   12.50
Coll. de docum. inéd. sur l'histoire de France. 53.

292. **Marine. — Sprout, H. and M.,** The rise of American naval power, 1776–1918. Princeton, 1939. W. map and pl. cloth.   7.50

293. — **Taylor, Ch. C.,** The life of Admiral Mahan, naval philosopher, Rear-admiral U.S. navy (1840–1914). London, 1920. Av. portr. et pl. toile. (12.60)   6.—

294. — **Van Tenac,** Histoire générale de la marine, compren. les naufrages célèbres, les voyages autour du monde, les découvertes et colonisations, l'histoire des pirates, corsaires et negriers, exploits des marins illustres, voyages dans les mers glaciales, guerres et batailles navales jusqu'au bombardement de Tanger et la prise de Mogador. Paris, Penaud frères, (1853). 4 vol. Av. 40 pl., grav. s. acier ou s. bois, dont 7 color., représent. des uniformes de la marine et des pavillons. d. veau.   30.—

295. — **Zeis, P. M.,** American shipping policy. Princeton, 1938. cloth. 6.—
„Why government subsidy has failed to produce a first-rate merchant marine".

296. **Mediterranean islands. — Wilstach, P.,** Islands of the Mediterranean. London, 1926. W. 31 pl. cloth. (9.60)   3.50
Majorca, Corsica, Elba, Malta, Sardinia, Corfu, Cyprus, etc. etc.

297. **Moravian brothers. — Le Long, I.,** Godts wonderen met zyne kerke,.... verhaal, van meest Boheemsche en Moravische Broeders, die.... een Evangel. Broeder-gemeente gesticht hebben, te Herrnhuth. 2e dr. verb. Amst., A. Wor en Erve G. onder de Linden, 1738 Av. vue sur Herrnhuth. pet. in-8vo. vél.   25.—
Histoire de la communion protestante des frères moraves ou „Hernhutters" qui descendent des disciples de Joh. Husz.
Chap. XV. Extract eener reys-beschryvinge, van Herrnhuth, over Coppenhagen, naar St. Thomas in America, en wederom terug, 1732–1733. — Chap. XVI. Idem naar Groenlandt, van drie timmerlieden, 1733.

298. **Netherlands: Topography and history. — Aa, C. P. E. Robidé van der,** Oud-Nederland in de uit vroegere dagen overgeblevene burgen en kasteelen geschetst en afgebeeld. Nijmegen, 1846. Av. 72 pl. lith. gr. in-8vo. d.veau. (Dos endomm.).   35.—
Un des meilleurs ouvrages sur les vieux chateaux dans les Pays-Bas. Epuisé et rare.

299. — **Allan, F.,** Het eiland Vlieland en zijne bewoners. Amst. 1857. W. map.   3.—

300. — **Baerdt van Sminia, H.,** Nieuwe naamlijst van grietmannen van de vroegste tijden tot 1795. M. aanteek. Leeuwarden, 1837. — **A. J. Andreae,** Nalezing op de Nieuwe naamlijst. Leeuwarden, 1893. — Ens. 2 vol. cart.   10.—

301. — **Bouman, J.,** Bedijking, opkomst en bloei van de Beemster. Purmerende, 1857. Av. portrait de Dirck van Oss et 3 cartes.   6.—

302. — **Bijdragen tot de geschiedenis van Overijsel.** Zwolle, 1874–1907. Série I, 10 vol. et 2 tables; série II, t. I–IV. Ens. 16 tom. 15 vol. d.rel.   60.—
Tout ce qui a paru. La seconde série est rare.

Prices are in guilders

303. **Netherlands. — Bijdragen tot de oudheidkunde en geschiedenis, in-
zonderh. van Zeeuwsch Vlaanderen.** Verz. d. H. Q. Janssen en J.
H. van Dale. Middelburg, 1856–63. 6 vol. 40.—
Collection complète. Recueil très estimé, conten. une quantité d'articles
sur l'histoire politique et ecclésiast., les antiquités religieuses et profanes,
les privilèges, octrois, sentences, etc. de la Flandre-Zélandaise.

304. **— Ceremonieboek** van de regeering van Amsterdam. (Amst. 1750).
Av. 3 pl., indiquant les places des bourgmestres, échevins etc.
lors des sessions offic. fol. d.veau. 10.—
Donne des particularités intéressantes sur les différ. cérémonies qui
eurent lieu à l'occasion des élections de nouveaux bourgmestres, de membres de la municipalité, de membres du tribunal, etc.

305. **— Van Dedem. — Requesten** en stukken van Jonkheer Willem Carel
van Dedem, relatief tot desselfs admissie als ampts jonker 's ampts
eede, in de provintie van Gelderland, quartier van Veluwe, nef-
fens vier advisen en een conformatoir van neutrale Geldersche
regtsgeleerden. Arnhem, J. Nijhoff, 1775. pet. in-fol. d.veau.
Très rare. 10.—

306. **— Dorsman, K.,** De ambachtsheerlijkheid Rijswijk voorheen en
thans. (Rijswijk, 1909). Av. 30 ill. Rel. en soie blanche. 1.50

307. **— Dutch, The,** drawn to the life. London, 1664. W. front. sm. 8vo.
Russia. 36.—
Contains: A description of Holland and the Dutch provinces of the
civill government of the United Provinces. The Dutch customes. The
private qualities, condition and carriage of the Dutch. Our right to
the Narrow Seas. The inestimable benefit the Dutch make of the British
Seas. The lives and characters of the princes of Aurange.
The front. and the titlepage margined.

308. **— Geul, I.,** Delfs-Haeghsche tweedracht, verandert in een-macht.
Voor ghestelt over het maken vande Haeghsche vaert, nae het
West-landt, ende de Delfsche proceduren daer tegens. 's Grav.,
A. J. Tongerloo, 1644. 4to. 7.50
Not in Knuttel. Van der Wulp, no. 2711.

309. **— Goossen Jzn., G.,** Geschiedkundige en plaatselijke beschrijving
van Wageningen. Wageningen, 1862. Av. 2 pl. d.veau. *Rare.* 6.—

310. **— Guibal, C. J.,** Democratie en oligarchie in Friesland tijdens
de Republiek. Assen, 1934. (3.90) 2.—

311. **— Heeringa, K.,** Beschrijving van Schiedam. I. Schiedam vóór
1600. Schiedam, 1910. Av. plan color. d'après van Deventer et
12 ill. gr. in-fol. 5.—
Tout ce qui a paru.

312. **— (Kindermann, J. C.),** Lodewijk van Nassau, de volmaakte
ridder, 1538–1574. Utrecht, 1874. 1.—

313. **— Kuin Jr., P.,** Het eiland Marken. Groningen, 1932. W. ill. (1.90)
1.—
Studiën op het gebied van ethnologie, etc. I.

314. **— Lutgers, P. J.,** Gezigten in de omstreken van Utrecht. M. geschiedkund. aanteek. van W. J. Hofdijk. S. l. 1869. Av. 87 belles
pl. lithograph. fol. En portef. 90.—

315. **— Magnin, J. S.,** Losse bladen uit Drenthe's geschiedenis. Assen,
1856. 4.50
Het branden van Meivuren in Drenthe verboden, 1663. — De laatste
wolvejagten in Drenthe. — etc.

316. **Netherlands. — Nieuwenhuys, C. J.**, Proeve eener geneeskundige
plaatsbeschrijving (topographie) der stad Amsterdam. Amst., J.
van der Hey, 1816–20. 4 vol. Av. grands plans et de nombr. tabl.
d. rel. *Très rare.*   20.—
      Karakter der Amsterdammers. — Leefwijze en kleeding, spijs en drank.
      — Nijverheid en zakelijkheid der A. — Vermaken. — Bevolking, geboorte
      en sterfte. — Geneeskundig onderwijs. — Ziekten. — Begraven. — Toe-
      stand en onderstand der gezonde armen. — Over de zieke armen. — Gast-
      huizen. — Sterfte der zieken. — Verzorging der armen. — Weeshuizen. —
      Gevangenen en gevangenissen. — Policie. — Geneeskundige wetten.

317. **— Nijhoff, I. A.**, Gedenkwaardigheden uit de geschiedenis van
Gelderland, door onuitgegeven oorkonden opgehelderd. Arnhem,
's-Grav. 1830–75. 6 vols. in 8. 4to.   85.—
      History of Gelderland, from the beginning of the 14th century till the
      year 1535, with numerous unpublished charters, documents, etc.
      Out of print and much sought after.

318. **— Oera Linda Bok, Thet**, naar een hs. uit de 13e eeuw. Met ver-
gunning van C. Over de Linden, bewerkt, vert. en uitgeg. d. J.
C. Ottema. Leeuwarden, 1872. W. 1 pl. and 2 facs. hfbound. *Rare.*
                                                                            18.—
      Added: **Ottema, J. G.**, Geschiedkund. aanteek. en ophelder. bij Thet Oera
      Linda Bok. 1873.

319. **— Oltmans, A.**, De gemeente Assen in hare wording en ontwikkeling. Assen, 1907. Av. pl.   1.50

319a. **— Placcaert** vande Staten generael vande gheunieerde Nederlanden, byden welcken, ... men verclaert den Coninck van
Spaegnien vervallen vande overheyt ende heerschappije van dese
voors. Nederlanden. Leyden, Ch. Silvius, 1581. 24 pp. 4to. hfcalf.
                                                                            50.—
      Tiele, nr. 236. O r i g i n a l e d i t i o n, e x t r e m e l y s c a r c e, of
      the famous Act of Abjuration of king Philip II of Spain by the States
      General of the Netherlands, July 26th 1581.
      F i n e, v e r y c l e a n c o p y, w i t h w i d e m a r g i n s. The copy
      has the last blank leaf, on the v° of which, in contempor. ms.: Gepubliceert
      te Bruessele den lesten dach van Augusto A° XVCLXXXI by W? Van....
      broeck.

320. **— Spaen, W. A. van**, Historie van Gelderland. Utrecht, 1814.
T. I (seul paru). d.veau.   17.50
      Histoire du duché de Gueldre jusqu'à 1343. Très rare.

321. **— Stads- en dorpskroniek** van Friesland, 1700–1900. (Uitgeg.)
d. G. A. Wumkes. Leeuwarden, 1930, 34. 2 vol. Av. reprod. d'an-
ciennes grav. dans le texte. (15.—)   10.—

322. **— Stukken** voor de vaderlandsche historie, (1555–1592). Uitgeg. d.
G. van Hasselt. Arnhem, W. Troost en Zoon, 1792–93. 4 vol. 17.50
      Recueil très intéressant, conten. des documents sur l'histoire des trou-
      bles dans la prov. de Gueldre. Une continuation se trouve dans les ,, Bijdra-
      gen voor vaderl. geschied. en oudheidkunde." (Série I, III, 29, 184 ss.).

323. **— Veegens, D.**, Historische studiën. Uitgeg. d. J. D. Veegens.
's-Grav. 1884. 2 vol.   4.50

324. **— Veen, S. D. van**, Historische studiën en schetsen. Groningen,
1905. toile. (4.90)   2.75
      Contient e.a.: De menuet en de domineespruik. — Innerlijk leven der
      vaderlandsche kerk in de 17e eeuw. — Een boeteprediker. — Foecke
      Floris. — Abr. Trommius. — De studie der theologie te Groningen in de 1e
      helft der 18e eeuw. — etc.

Prices are in guilders

325. **Netherlands. — Volksoverleveringen, Nederlandsche.** Verz. en met aanteek. d. J. W. Wolf. Bew. en m. bijv. verm. I: Friesland. Groningen, 1844. 1.25

326. **— Vries, R. W. P. de,** Amsterdamsche stadsgezichten. Amst. 1913. pet. in-fol. 1.—
Description des 20 vues connues sur la ville d' A. des 16e et 17e siècles.

327. **— Water, J. W. te,** Historie van het verbond en de smeekschriften der Nederl. edelen, 1565–1567. Middelburg, 1776–96. 4 vol. d. veau. *Bel ex.* 12.—
Le t. I en 2e édition.

328. **— Witt, P. de,** Une invasion prussienne en Hollande en 1787. Paris, 1886. 12mo. d. veau. 1.25

329. **— Wolf, K.,** Des Grafen Johann von Nassau Bemühungen um die Niederländischen Flüchtlinge. 's-Grav. 1935. *T. à p.* 1.—
— See also: **House of Orange. — Margaret of Austria.**

330. **Nijhoff, M.,** Het verhaal van den vos. Eene vroolijke vertooning met zang en dans. N. h. Russisch van I. Strawinsky. Amst. 1933. 1.—

331. **(Osborne, J.),** The problem of Japan. By an ex-counsellor of legation in the Far East. Amst. 1918. 5.—

332. **Papal bulls. — Adrianus Florentinus VI,** Regule, ordinationes et constitutiones Cancellariae.... Adriani papae. Antverpiae, Michel Hillenius, 1522, 16 Dec.
Nijhoff-Kronenberg, no. 11.
— — Regule Cancellarie nove: Super totali revocatione Expectativarum etc. Antverpiae, Mich. Hillenius, 1523. 2 Jan.
Nijhoff-Kronenberg, no. 2234. Sheet G. only. (Corresponds with the above).
— **Bulla** induciarum s. treugarum triennalium inter omnes Christianos reges et principes per Adrianum VI. No pl. (1523).
— **Clemens VII,** Regule, ordinationes et constitutiones.... Clementis papae VII.... Antverp., Mich. Hillenius, 1523, 24 Dec.
Bound up with:
— **Bulle Sacri Concilii Lateranensis.** (1513–1517). Romae, Steph. Guillereti, 1517. 8 pieces.
Collection of 8 papal bulls referring to the above.
In 1 vol. sm.8vo. calf. 60.—
Here and there some scratches.

333. **Perk, M. A.,** Schetsen en beelden. Haarlem, 1900. Av. portr. 1.75
Een etmaal in een trappistenklooster. — Palestijnsche herinneringen. — De Weselsche feesten 7 Aug. 1896. — Een voorlooper en wegbereider van Griekenland's wedergeboorte. — etc.

334. **Pleysier, A.,** De mensch in de leerschool van moeder aarde. Overzicht van de aardrijkskundige factoren die invloed hebben uitgeoefend op de ontwikkeling der volken. Amst. 1931. Av. cartes, pl. et ill. (735 pp.). (10.50) 4.50

335. **Polak, J. J.,** Publieke werken als vorm van conjunctuurpolitiek. 's-Grav. 1938. 3.20

336. **Poland. — Actes,** éditées par la Commission impériale (*plus tard:*) de Wilna, pour la recherche d'actes anciens de Wilna, 1388–1889. (Texte russe). Wilna, 1865–1915. 39 tom. 38 vol. 4to. dont 8 vol. d. veau, le reste en livr. 700.—
Plusieurs pièces en latin et en polonais.
Tout ce qui a paru.

Mart. Nijhoff, The Hague — Cat. No. 630

337. **Poland. — Fisher, H. H.,** and **S. Brooks,** America and the new
Poland. N. York, 1928. Av. cartes. toile. (8.25)   2.50

338. **— Linde, Van der,** Leven en daaden van Joh. Sobieski de III,
koning van Polen; mitsg. allen voorgaande Poolsche en Hunga-
rische koningen. Amst. 1685. 3 vols. in 1. W. front., plan and 9 pl.
4to. vellum.   40.—
      A very valuable work on the life of Johan Sobieski, Poland's greatest
      king.

339. **— Rutten, F.,** Polen. Een herboren land. 's-Grav. 1931. Av. pl.
(3.75)   1.50

340. **Priesthood. — Lippert, J.,** Allgemeine Geschichte des Priester-
thums. Berlin, 1883, 84. 2 vol. d. rel.   12.—

341. **— Louw, S. W.,** Het ontstaan van het priesterschap in de Christe-
lijke kerk. Utrecht, 1892.   1.25

342. **Prostitution. — Wilson, C. G.,** Chinatown quest. The life and
adventures of Donaldina Cameron. Stanford University, 1931.
Av. portrait et 7 pl. toile.   5.25
      „The story of Donaldina Cameron's life-long battle to end the traffic
      in Chinese slave-girls in this country (California) is here told for the first
      time.

343. **Quakers. — Bedrieger, De groote,** ondersocht ofte leven, onder-
soeck en ondervraging van James Naylor, de verleyde en ver-
leydende Quaker met de wijse van sijn inrijdingh binnen Bristol.
Na de copye van London, 1657. 4to.   7.50

344. **— Bourrough, E.,** Een standaert opgerecht, ende een baniere
voorgehouden tot alle natien.... door duysenden van sijn volck..
in spot Quaeckers genaemt. 3e dr. Amst., Chr. Cunradus, 1669. 4to.
                                                             10.—
      Maximes de la secte religieuse des Quakers.

345. **— Duivel, De,** verandert in een Quaeker ofte de verdoemlijke....
leeringen.... van die booze bedriegers, genaamt Quaekers, enz.
U.h. Eng. Utrecht, 1657. 4to.   1.50

346. **— Sewel, W.,** Histori van de opkomste, aanwas en voortgang
der Christenen, bekend bij den naam van quakers. M. authent.
stukken. Amst., R. en G. Wetstein, 1717. fol. Hfcalf. (840 pp.).
                                                             35.—
      Original edition of this wellknown standard work. Sewel spent 25 years
      in preparing his work on „The history of the rise, increase and progress of
      the Christian people called Quakers". The English edition, transl. by Sewel
      himself from Dutch into English appeared 1722. Sewel's work was based
      upon a mass of correspondence and its accuracy has never been impugned.
      The work is full of American interest containing also the history of the Qua-
      kers in New Netherland, Virginia, etc.

347. **Railways. — Chemin de fer, Le,** du Yunnan (par la Cie française
des chemins de fer de l'Indo-Chine et du Yunnan, etc.). Paris,
1910. 1 vol. de texte av. pl. en couleurs et en noir et 1 vol. de 55
cartes et plans, dont plusieurs se dépliant. fol. d. veau.   35.—

348. **— Congrès internat., 3e,** des chemins de fer. Paris 1889. Compte
rendu général. Brux. 1890. 3 vol. 4to. d. veau.   22.—

349. **— —** Idem, 4e. St. Pétersbourg 1892. Compte rendu général.
Brux. 1893, 94. 4 vol. 4to.   25.—

                    Prices are in guilders

350. **Railways.** — **Congrès internat., 5e,** des chemins de fer. Londres 1895. Compte rendu général. Brux. 1896–97. 4 vol. 4to.   24.—
Ajouté: Compte rendu sommaire.

351. — — Idem, 6e. Paris 1900. Compte rendu général. Brux. 1901, 02. 6 vol. 4to.   36.—

352. — — Idem, 7e. Washington 1905. Compte rendu général. Brux. 1906. 3 vol. Av. pl., figg. et tabl. 4to. d. rel.   15.—

353. — — Idem, 8e. Berne 1910. Compte rendu. Brux. 1911. 2 vol. 4to. veau espagnol.   24.—

354. — **Congrès, 13e,** (de l') Association internat. des chemins de fer. Paris 1937. Rapports. Brux. (1937, 38). 4to. In parts.   17.50
Publ. aussi dans Bulletin de l'Association internat. du Congrès des chemins de fer.

355. — **Congrès internat., 19e,** de tramways, de chemins de fer d'intérêt local et de transports publics automobiles. Paris 1924. Comptes rendus détaillés. Brux. 1925. Av. de nombr. cartes et figg. 4to. *Épuisé.*   15.—

356. — — Idem, 20e. Barcelone 1926. Comptes-rendus. Brux. 1926. 4to.   18.—

357. — — Idem, 23e. La Haye 1932. Comptes-rendus. Brux. 1932. 4to.   27.50

358. — — Idem, 24e. Berlin 1934. [Rapports]. Brux. 1934. 4to. 30.—

359. — — Idem, 25e. Vienne 1937. Comptes rendus. [Rapports]. Brux. 1938. 4to.   50.—
The text of 6 of the reports is in german.

360. — **Cordier, J.,** Considérations sur les chemins de fer. Paris, 1830. Av. 2 cartes et 1 pl. couv. orig.   90.—
De toute rareté, avec les cartes et planches (Plan de la route en fer de Liverpool à Manchester; Machines locom. Le Sans-Pareil, La Nouveauté, Le Rocket; Carte du projet d e l i g n e d e B a l t i m o r e à l'O h i o). One of the earliest works in French on railroads. The author gives a survey of the English and American inventions and projects.

361. — **Goschler, Ch.,** Traité pratique de l'entretien et de l'exploitation des chemins de fer. 2e éd. Paris, 1870, 72. 2 vol. Av. figg. et un Atlas de 35 pl. Ens. 3 vol. d. mar.   5.—

362. — **Kongress, 22er Internat.,** der Strassenbahnen, Kleinbahnen und der öffentl. Kraftfahrtunternehmen. Warschau 1930. Ausführl. Bericht. Brüssel, 1931. 4to.   25.—

363. — — Idem, 23er. Haag 1932. Ausführl. Bericht. Brüssel, 1933. 4to.   27.50

364. — **Perdonnet, A.,** Traité élément. des chemins de fer. 3e éd. Paris, 1865. 4 vol. Av. portr., cartes, pl. et ill. d. rel.   10.—
Contient e.a.: Histoire et statistique des chemins de fer (Europe, Amérique septentr., Amérique méridion., Afrique, Asie, Océanie). — De l ı disposition des gares. — Théorie des locomotives. — etc.

365. — **Raab, C. J.,** Special-Karte der Eisenbahn-, Post- und Dampfschiff-Verbindungen Mittel-Europa's. Mit Angabe.... der Grenzen des Zollvereins. Gezeichnet von H. Muller. Glogau, (v. 1865). Carte collée sur toile, mes. 1.35 × 1.18 M. En étui.   2.50

366. — **Seguin Ainé,** De l'influence des chemins de fer et de l'art de les tracer et de les construire. Paris, 1839. Av. 6 pl. de figg. d. veau. 45.—
Important and scarce work by this great scientist and engineer. First edition.

367. **Railways. — Teisserenc, E.,** De la politique des chemins de fer et
de ses applications diverses. Paris, 1842. 2 vol. Av. 2 cartes.   12.—
   Travail important d'un ingénieur à qui on doit de nombr. études techni-
   ques sur la rivalité des chemins de fer et des canaux, les pentes, etc. Rare.

368. **— Wiener, L.,** L'Egypte et ses chemins de fer. Brux. 1932. Av.
portraits et 272 cartes, ill. et figg.   15.—
   Cet ouvrage présente d'abord une étude sur le régime du Nil. Il étudie
   ensuite les chemins de fer de l'Etat, reprenant leur développement jusqu'à
   ce jour et l'examen de chacun des grands départements: Voies et travaux
   — Ponts — Traction et matériel roulant — Administration et exploitation. De la même façon il étudie les autres compagnies égyptiennes de
   chemins de fer.
   C'est pour la première fois que l'on a réuni un ensemble de ce genre.

369. **— Wood, N.,** A practical treatise on rail-roads and interior com-
munication in general. Containing an account of the performan-
ces of the different locomotive engines at and subsequent to the
Liverpool contest; upwards of 260 experiments, etc. London,
1831. Av. 11 pl. et 1 tabl. d. veau.   25.—

370. **Rhætian Bible, etc. — Bibla, La sacra,** quai ais tuotla Sancta Scrit-
türa. Tschantada, vertida è stampada in lingua Rumanscha d'Inga-
dinna Bassa; tras cumün cuost è larvûr da J. A. Vulpio et J. Dorta
à Vulpera. Scuol in Ingadina Bassa tras J. Dorta a Vulpera, 1679.
4 parts in 1 strong vol. fol. oak boards, covered with blind tooled
leather, edges and clasps in copper.   75.—
   The first product from the presses, established by Jacques Dorta a
   Vulpera at Scuoll, little community in the Swiss canton of the Grisons.
   This translation of the Bible in the Rhaetian language is very scarce. It
   consists of 4 parts, each one with a separate title; that of the 3d part is
   decorated by a large woodcut-border with biblical personages, that of the
   1st part seems to be missing. However there is the general title, which
   precedes the whole.
   A spot on the general title; one leaf and the margine of the last three
   leaves repaired; otherwise in good condition.

371. **— Cudesch da Psalms, Un,** chi suun fatts è miss da chiantar in Ladin,
ils quaus sum impart eir uyuaunt flatts luguads da chiantar in
Tudaischk, ed impart brichia, etc. Tuot tratt aqui insemmel in un
csarpe dritzad a chiantar in Romaunsch, traas Durich Chiampel.
Basel, in chiasa de Jachiam Kündig, 1562. pet. in-8vo. veau ancien.   35.—
   A la fin: Vn intraguida maint dad infurmar la Giuuantün in la uaira
   cretta, etc. Traas D. Chiampell.
   Première édition de la traduction rhétique des Psaumes, e x t r ê m e-
   m e n t   r a r e, un des premiers ouvrages imprimés en langue rhétoromane.
   Ex. dans un état peu frais ayant qq. ff. restaurés comme tous les livres
   de ce genre. Au commencement 10 ff. sont en facs. ainsi que le dernier f.
   En outre il y manque les pp. 15/16 et 21-32 de l'introduction, les pp.
   271/72 du texte et le f. Nn, 7 du dernier ouvrage. A la page 318 se trouve
   une marque d'imprimeur ainsi qu'une autre à la p. 512. Le f. blanc entre
   les pp. 318 et 321 s'y trouve.

372. **— Testamaint, L'gnouf Saench,** da .... Jesu Christi, prais our delg
Latin et our d'oters languaigs, e huossa da noef mis in Arumaunsch,
traes Jachiam Biffrun d'Agnedina. Puschlaeff, Dolfin et Dolfin
Landolfs, 1607. XXXII and 911 pp. sm. 8vo. old calf.   40.—
   Rhaetian translation, extremely scarce, of the New Testament. The first
   edition was publ. in 1560.
   The titlepage and the last 2 ll. in beautiful facs., pp. 455-458 missing.
   Some spots. Back slightly damaged.